The Fundame

The Fundamentals of Ear Acupuncture

By Helmut Kropej, M. D.

Translated by Diana Reese-Soltész

With 38 Figures and 7 Tables

4th edition

Karl F. Haug Publishers · Heidelberg

Deutsche Bibliothek Cataloguing-in-Publication Data

Kropej, Helmut:
The fundamentals of ear acupuncture / by Helmut Kropej. Transl. by Diana Reese-Soltész.
– 4. ed. – Heidelberg : Haug, 1991
   Dt. Ausg. u.d.T.: Kropej, Helmut: Systematik der Ohrakupunktur
   ISBN 3-7760-0777-X

2nd edition 1984
3rd edition 1987
4th edition 1991

Title-No. 1777 · ISBN 3-7760-0777-X

Printed in West-Germany by Progressdruck GmbH, 6720 Speyer

CONTENTS

FOREWORD

This book is the result of an endeavour to present ear acupuncture*) in the systematic form to which the Western-trained physician is accustomed.

Until quite recently, reflex therapy via the ear merely represented a supplement to the therapeutic palette of a small number of physicians. However, it is slowly becoming an established therapeutic method and the number of doctors interested in it is continuously increasing.

I have tried to find a compromise between a simple interpretation, which is tempting to the beginner (and in which some of the complicated theory of auricular therapy remains in the background) and the treatment method used at present. This endeavour is in accord with the Vienna School of Acupuncture as represented by the Ludwig Boltzmann Acupuncture Institute.

Therefore, I have tried to limit myself mainly to the description of those zones and points which have proven themselves effective to me and my colleagues at the institute and in private practice. We feel that speculations that some of the organism's most complicated areas project to the auricle according to anatomical viewpoints alone, having no statistical foundation, seem just as suspicious to a physician as does the idea that every thinkable emotion has its own reflex point.

The members of the Ludwig Boltzmann Acupuncture Institute, guided by its director, Prof. Johannes *Bischko,* M. D., have taken it upon themselves, with the aid of other scientific institutes, to statistically establish the individual reflex areas on the ear and to study their effect in the laboratory. The results of this research can be found in special articles in medical and scientific publications.

This book deals with auricular therapy in the practical sense only. I have not dealt with questions which, on the basis of our present knowledge, must still remain unanswered. I have made no

---

*) Ear acupuncture is also called auriculo or auricular therapy, in other languages as well, such as German, French, Italian, and Spanish.

attempt to present new theoretical explanations of the way ear acupuncture works. Unfortunately, all theories which have been published up to now have produced no working hypotheses and are all based on long-recognized neurophysiological facts. These theories have yet to be proven scientifically. In my opinion, experimental proof should be established on an interdisciplinary level and confined to scientific institutes.

A great number of English-speaking colleagues come to our institute to observe and study. A frequently-heard complaint was that they were unable to find any suitable literature on ear acupuncture in English, therefore, I decided to have an English version of my (originally German-language) book published. My book is based on *Nogier's* most certainly correct concepts which I did not find necessary to significantly change. The Vienna School is known for a certain conservatism, which has proven itself beneficial to both patients and physicians alike. This book is the simple result of many years of serious work. May it serve you well.

I would like to close this foreword by thanking my friends whose advice greatly helped me, in particular Prof. J. *Bischko,* who introduced me to acupuncture and supported me with his great experience. Very special thanks go to my wife who did all the written work for the original German-language version.

I would like to express my gratitude to Barnett *Junker,* M. D., Elfriede *Brauneis,* L. A. C. S. T., E. *Warth,* M. D., and Alec *Savicky,* M. D. for their thorough review of the rough drafts of the English manuscript, and especially to Diana *Reese-Soltész* who conscientiously translated my book into English with great care and attention to detail.

Vienna, May, 1979

Helmut *Kropej,* M. D.

FOREWORD TO THE SECOND EDITION

The development of reflex therapy via the ear has taken leaps and bounds in the last few years. Alone the gradual change in how this form of therapy is named reflects this fact.

Originally termed ear acupuncture, the name auricular medicine was adopted upon the discovery of the so-called RAC or *Nogier's* reflex, containing auricular diagnosis and auricular therapy. In 1978, the term "New Medicine of Energy" was coined, presumably to stress the self-reliance of this therapy. Medicine therewith became another new "system" richer. There have always been a lot of systems in medicine, for example, the old humoral medicine, neural therapy, or homoeopathy. They were all only partially successful, and academic medicine assimilated their assets to only a limited degree. However, at least their basic concepts were taken note of, and obscure misusage, in contrast, abandoned. There are two main hindrances to real growth of a basic idea which pave the way for mysticism and lead to a fringe existence: 1. imprudent striving for constant renewal, and 2. indiscriminate credulity. It goes without saying that no science remains static, but is in continual flow. This applies not only to formal and empirical science, but also to science in its simplest form (collecting, describing, and classifying facts). But the asserted hypotheses must always remain in suitable relation to the duration of their validity. It is easier to make suggestive claims than to give exact proof. Sensational claims attract more attention, and, if convincingly presented, even erroneous single observations tend to be more readily accepted than painstaking refutations and scrutiny (Le Bon). In science, however, one should always be conscious of the level on which the contemplations and actions in question are taking place.

Spectacular as they may at times be, single observations are best passed over in silence, especially when they can neither be explained nor reproduced in a significant manner. Only with reproducible results, the explanation of which does not contradict the classical foundations of medicine to too great a degree, can a method not yet accepted by academic medicine find its place therein.

The second edition of this book has been revised and improved in keeping with the contemplations expressed and discussed in various seminars and at our institute.

Vienna, May, 1984   Helmut *Kropej,* M. D.

INTRODUCTION

More than twenty years have gone by since Dr. P. *Nogier,* of Lyon, France, first reported on his "personal experiences with reflex zones and reflex points on the outer ear and auricle" during an acupunture congress in Marseille. Within one year (1957), G. *Bachmann*'s German translation of this speech, which appeared in the "Deutsche Zeitschrift für Akupunktur", had already captured the interest of a large number of physicians. Since then, ear acupuncture has continued to grow in significance in the West and East alike.

It is difficult to say with certainty in which country stimulating the auricle for therapeutic purposes originated. Records exist which show that the Chinese studied the ear and its relation to the rest of the body long before our chronology begins. The ear also seems to be the center of the meridian system in traditional Chinese medicine. All Yang and Yin meridians are closely related to the ear via partner meridians (i. e. Lung-Large Intestine). Indications for reflex therapy via the ear were already recorded in the first centuries A. D. *Schnorrenberger* mentions the "A shi" point in the Chinese primer, "A Thousand Precious Prescriptions". This refers to treatment of points on the edge of the ear which are sensitive to pressure. "A", says the Chinese patient when the painful spot is touched, and "Shi", when treatment of the point has brought relief.

Records made during the **T'ang Dynasty** (618—907) mention twenty anterior and posterior ear points. One of these is found in the auricle and probably corresponds with *Nogier*'s O-point. More information on the use of ear points exists in the Chinese literature.

The method probably travelled via trade routes and waterways from China to Africa, Persia, and India, and from there to the Mediterranean area. It seems to have survived longest in the South of France and North Africa, where treatment via the auricle consisted mainly of cauterization for relief of sciatica.

It was no doubt *Nogier*'s keen perception which led him to study more closely the observations he had made in his private practice. He detected scars on the ears of several of his patients, all on the same spot. They were the result of cauterization for relief of sciatic pain. The ingenious idea of connecting this area on the anthelix with the lumbo-sacral articulation and thus of the anthelix as the reflex area of the entire spinal column (however, upside-down, like an embryo in the womb) led to the reflex cartography of the ear.

The concept of a pathophysiological connection between the ear and the rest of the body is very old — it was reintroduced in 1739 by *WouK'ien* in "Yi-tsong kiu-kien", which illustrates the Chinese areas of projection of the body on the ear *(Jarricot)*. Still, I believe we may assume that *Nogier*'s intensive research and the systematic development of the method by the Chinese were decisive in proving the significance of ear acupuncture and in encouraging further development. Achieving analgesia via zones of the ear may represent the final stage at present of this development.

After this historical summary, I would now like to delve into the principles of auricular therapy in detail.

The following statement best describes the possibilities and limitations of auricular therapy:

"Auricular therapy is a treatment form in which points on the auricle which are sensitive to pressure and electrically measurable may be used for diagnosis or for treatment of various functional illnesses and disorders by means of manual, electrical, or other suitable stimulation."

The goal is to produce a change in the area or organ which has caused the corresponding point on the auricle to manifest itself. Here, change means functional normalization or, if pain is present, relief or alleviation.

The discovery of causal localizations in functional or organic disturbances through detection of altered points on a seemingly healthy auricle is of particular interest. In a healthy person, the skin of the auricle is normally painless. However, if a disorder exists, slightly painful points on the auricle can be detected. These sometimes make themselves noticeable (the so-called spontaneously painful points). Usually, however, they are found by examining the auricle with a bougie or probe. These painful points may correspond with affected regions of the body or functional disorders.

The point's alteration also makes itself evident via its electrical conductivity. Every point on the ear with a lowered resistance in comparison to the area immediately surrounding it is abnormal and corresponds with a pathological state in an organ or region.

Auricular therapy seems to me to be superior to body acupuncture for diagnosis because of the fact that the corresponding points of the ear only reveal themselves when a functional disturbance or illness exists in the body. Not only that, but close examination of the auricle itself may also provide valuable information as to the corresponding organ, especially in long-term illnesses. For example, in chronic illnesses, redness, scale formation, nodules, and ulcers can be found on the corresponding zone. The points within the corresponding zone are always closely connected with the **individual** anatomical relief of the auricle. This fact, and those mentioned above, make the use of points and point combinations according to standard programs impossible in ear acupuncture.

Mere knowledge of the ear points is insufficient for solving each individual problem with which you will be faced. You will only achieve success with this method if you have established the pathophysiological mechanisms of the disorder with which you are confronted and have made an exact analysis of the related pain. You will only be able to treat a specific case and effectively influence complicated disorders when you have comprehended the individual disorder in its entirety. This essentially distinguishes auricular therapy from Far Eastern data on the therapy of various disorders. As we will see later on, repeated use of the same point combination will never achieve adequate results.

Another difference is the Chinese attempt to combine ear acupuncture with their traditional medicine. Hence, in the "therapy program" of the Chinese ear acupuncture primer, we note that they have tried to include the organ theory of classical acupuncture. From the Chinese point of view, this may be theoretically justified, as the organ theory represents the basis of traditional Chinese medicine. Indeed, in the theory of traditional Chinese medicine, the term Dsang-Fu (the organ) denotes not only an anatomically defined organ, but also its physiological function. This may be of significance for body acupuncture. However, it is not only difficult for the Western auricular therapist to understand, but is also impractical, since auricular therapy only employs corresponding ear points which reveal themselves during an illness.

Let me give you a concrete example. A point of the zone corresponding with the kidneys has yet to become manifest if the patient is suffering from a bone disease. However, in the organ theory, the Kidney is "the Master of the Bones", and is closely related to bone growth and development. Hence, the attempt is made to orientalize auricular therapy.

I am of the opinion that the same reasons are responsible for this as for the Western world attempting to westernize traditional Chinese medicine. And just as Europe and the West are gradually finding their way back to the original concepts of traditional acupuncture, so in a few years, the Chinese may also begin using auricular therapy according to *Nogier*'s basic concept without combining it with their traditional concepts.

We all owe our thanks to Dr. P. F. M. *Nogier* of Lyon, France, whose keenness, joy of discovery, and endless diligence were responsible for expanding the therapeutic possibilities of medical treatment through auricular therapy.

The Correspondence Point

Just as in classical body acupuncture, the "point" is the focus of attention in auricular therapy. However, on the ear, these are physiologically altered points, which correspond with maximum points within corresponding zones. Whereas *Kellner* demonstrated accumulations of terminal structures with effector and receptor characteristics on body acupuncture points, histological studies performed hitherto on ear acupuncture points have shown no similar structures.

The ear acupuncture point will only be altered, sensitive to pressure, and electrically measurable when a peripheral disorder exists. Only some form of peripheral change, regardless of whether it involves a disturbed region, pain, or a functional disorder, will enable a latent point to be localized on a seemingly healthy auricle.

The following test will illustrate what I mean. It is based on the principle that a change in the sensitivity of a point of the auricle can be brought about by producing pain in the body. Before the test is commenced, the auricular area to be tested is examined with a bellied bougie or probe to make sure that no particular sensitivity already exists. Then the distal phalanx of the subject's thumb is pinched with a clamp. A few minutes later, the same area on the auricle is again tested for sensitivity with a bougie or probe. Even after this short interval, the subject will report a distinct change in sensitivity of a certain point. After several more minutes, this increases to such an extent that touching the point with the bougie is extremely painful and the subject grimaces, jerks his leg, or even cries out. Hence, the point corresponding to the phalanx of the thumb has been located.

Several minutes after the clamp has been removed, the point gradually loses its sensitivity until it is again completely indifferent to pressure.

One must, however, take note of the fact that the site of pain the patient describes need not necessarily coincide with the affected organ (transferred pain). The effect of pain stimuli on internal organs frequently does not at all lead to pronounced pain at the site of the affected organ, but rather to an indirect type of pain radiation resulting in pain in a superficial part of the body, this often far away from the site of the stimulus' action.

When referring to areas of the skin which are sensitive to pain, one speaks of Head's zones. Are deeper-lying structures or muscles and fibers affected, into which the visceral pain is transferred, they are termed Mackenzie's zones.

In auricular therapy, stimulation of the reflex zones of "transferred" pain localizations alone will not produce adequate results. These can only be achieved by stimulating the point of the organ actually causing pain. Painful conditions, therefore, necessitate sufficient analysis of the pain itself, this, however, requiring considerable pertinent knowledge.

As a rule, the auricle located on the same side of the body as the afflicted peripheral region contains the most information.

Therapy via the auricle uses the opposite process. Manual, electrical, or other suitable stimulation of the corresponding point on the auricle causes a change in the sensitivity or function of the related peripheral zone.

15

Although the points on the ear usually demonstrate lowered skin resistance, there are also some points whose resistance is higher than that of the skin surrounding them (in contrast to body points). Such points represent an "overabundance" of energy and must always be acupunctured with silver needles.

The above-described test clearly shows that the correspondence point of the auricle demonstrates unique specific behavior in that it is dependent on physiopathological factors, and again becomes "silent" when normalization of the peripheral conditions has been achieved. Aside from these points, which are characterized by a change in their vitality, there are others, which demonstrate **persistent physical characteristics.** That means they are always sensitive to pressure and can always be located by electrical means. These are correspondence points which are related to a chronic peripheral process or irreversible organic injury. These "permanent points" are helpful, for example, in locating vertebral or bone fractures having occurred long ago. They must frequently be included in the therapy program. Furthermore, there are also **spontaneously painful points** on the auricle. According to *Nogier,* "these represent a pathological aggression, and are not indicative of a negative prognosis". They should only be needled by experienced acupuncturists as they may release unpleasant reactions.

For practical reasons, the correspondence points are named after the regions of the body to which they correspond. Every physician likes to see either the indication or at least a hint of the chemical composition in the name of a new medication. Likewise, when confronted with a disorder in a peripheral region, he should be able to easily associate it with the reflex zone which has the same name as that region.

Locating the Points

This chapter gives an outline of the various methods of locating the correspondence points of the ear. It offers the basics for diagnosis and therapy via the auricle.

a) Examination of the Auricle

In the foregoing section on the correspondence point, I already mentioned that long-term or chronic disorders may cause pathological changes on the skin of the auricle. Hence, you may find reddened, point-formed areas, scales, swelling, and perhaps even small nodules in the corresponding region of the ear. You must pay special attention to these dermatological alterations. These points must always be included in the therapy program.

Because of the fact that the areas and points of the ear are closely related to the anatomical structure of the auricle, you must familiarize yourself with the anatomy of the entire auricle. Here, you must of course bear in mind that no two individuals have identical ear shapes, nor are both ears of the same person necessarily alike. Furthermore, as a person grows older, his auricle changes not only as far as elasticity and relief are concerned (more wrinkles), but also in regard to the relationships between the individual relief formations. This is of particular importance when determining the size of the individual correspondence zones.

b) Manual Detection of the Points

This subjective method is dependent on the patient's sensitivity and is used to determine the correspondence points' sensitivity to pressure. A special instrument has been designed for this purpose.

The PROBE designed according to *Nogier* has a relatively blunt point with a diameter of 1 mm^2 located on a spring in a metal cylinder. The spring tension is variable and corresponds to a pressure of 120—150 g when the point is retracted as far as possible. Any other bellied bougie is just as suitable.

The probe should always be held perpendicular to the skin surface. Hence, the probe is placed on the zone and the pressure is gradually increased. At the same time, the patient must be carefully observed as to reactions such as blinking, grimacing, etc.

Simple as this method is, it has the disadvantage of being dependent on the patient's subjective information. However, with more experience, the examiner will be able to surmount certain problems inherent in this method.

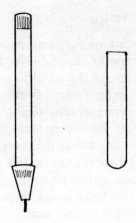

Fig. 1: Probe and "Stirrup"

c) Electrical Detection of Points

This is an objective method of examination independent of subjective information and reactions on the part of the patient. All point detectors on the market are based on the fact that acupuncture points demonstrate altered skin resistance.

I myself have been using the PUNCTOSCOPE*) exclusively for many years. This device was designed according to *Nogier's* data.

Like all other similar models, this apparatus sends a very weak current of about 20 μA, which has no therapeutic effect, to the body by means of a handle which represents the ground electrode. The reduced or increased skin resistance at the points is measured with a probe electrode.

In the Punctoscope, the probe electrode consists of 2 positively poled electrodes, one of which is rod-shaped. The other is cylindrical and encloses the rod-shaped electrode. Both are mounted independently on springs and are isolated rendering a short-circuit impossible. Only the ends of both electrodes are conductive. Contact of the rod electrode with the skin surface is made by means of a point; that of the cylinder electrode with a circle. This double electrode makes evaluation of the point's resistance in comparison to

*) Punctoscope, S.E.D.A.T. Company, France.

18

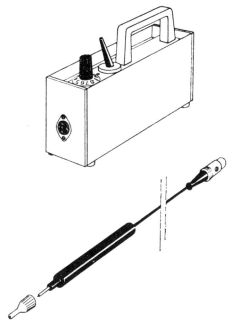

Fig. 2: The Punctoscope

that of the skin surrounding it possible. Hence, the absolute resistance of the point is not measured, but rather the relative resistance
in comparison to the surrounding skin. The device measures this
differential by means of a bridge circuit in which the rod electrode's value is compared with that of the cylinder electrode. A difference of about 4—5 µA is required for a positive measurement result. If a point has been found which demonstrates these criteria, a
buzzing signal sounds. It goes without saying that the device must
be adjusted to the lowest individual sensitivity by means of a potentiometer before point-location is commenced. With the potentiometer, the differential measurement between the rod and cylinder electrodes may be regulated. Here, turning the potentiometer
clockwise increases the device's sensitivity; the difference between
the rod and cylinder electrodes is reduced and thus, too many
points are found. This must be avoided. If the knob of the potentiometer is turned counterclockwise, the device becomes less sensi-

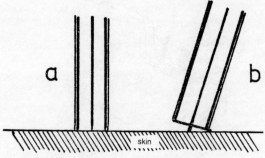

Fig. 3: Position of the probe electrode (receiver) of the Punctoscope on the skin surface. a) correct, applied perpendicularly, b) incorrect

tive, and the acoustic signal only sounds when there is a greater difference in resistance between the point and the surrounding skin.

Aside from the graduated potentiometer knob, the Punctoscope also has another small lever. When this lever is switched, the device can also detect points which demonstrate increased resistance in comparison to the surrounding skin. This additional function facilitates the selection of the metal of the needles to be used. Points which demonstrate a weak resistance require treatment with gold or molybdenum needles. Here, the little lever must be turned towards the notch on the Punctoscope. Points with a stronger resistance than the surrounding skin must be acupunctured with silver needles. To find these points, the lever must be turned away

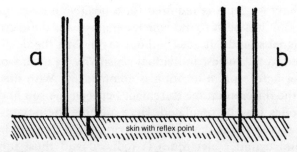

Fig. 4: a) Probe electrode near a reflex point of the auricle (the Punctoscope's buzzing tone is **inconstant**), b) Probe electrode on the center of the point (the buzzing tone is constant)

from the notch. Most of the points found on the ear are "gold points", hence, one must always commence examination of the ear with the lever turned towards the notch.

When using this device, you must be certain that the probe electrodes are applied perpendicularly to the skin surface, that they are only slightly pressed down, that is, 1—2 mm, and that the acoustic signal is constant. If the signal is interrupted, the point is either unstable, or you are close to the point, but the rod electrode is not on the point's center. If you have found a reflex point, press the retractable end of the probe down onto the skin to exactly mark the point.

Because of the fact that ear points are usually only 0.1 mm in size, an electronic point detector is necessary for therapy via the auricle.

The real prerequisite for correct point detection on the ear is patience on the part of the examiner. Systematic examination of the areas in question is the only way to achieve the desired results. Here, the saying "less is more" is valid. In other words, finding fewer but more effective points with a device adjusted to the patient's individual sensitivity is more important than finding many points which lead to inadequate results.

The Procedure of Point Detection

After taking down an exact medical history and having performed a thorough examination, you must determine the symptoms and cause of the disorder with which you are dealing, in order to determine which areas must be examined. Then, the patient must grasp the handle of the Punctoscope and push the lever towards the handle with his thumb to switch the device on. The examiner holds the probe electrode in his hand. Point detection is now commenced with the little lever switched towards the "notch" ("gold setting"). Adjusting the device according to individual sensitivity and laterality of the O-point used to be recommended. This is, however, no longer valid, as experience has shown that the O-point itself, which was formerly used as point of reference, may also be pathologically altered. Therefore, the more practical procedure is to commence point detection with the probe electrode applied perpendicularly to the skin surface and pressed down only slightly. The potentiometer should be adjusted to 5 or 6. If you have found a point which releases the buzzer even when the potentiometer is switched to 4, 3, or even 2, then you can be certain of having found a main point. If you have been unable to find an active point in the area where you expect to find it with the lever switched towards the notch, you must switch the lever in the opposite direction ("silver setting") and repeat the detection procedure. The signal is only significant when it remains constant.

You must always bear in mind that the size of the "points" varies greatly and may range from 0.1 to several mm². The size of the points or areas corresponds to the extent of the peripheral pathological process. Accordingly, you will have to use more needles for larger areas (e. g. for disorders of the knee, shoulder joint, or large intestine, etc.).

The device is relatively easy to use. Nevertheless, you must be familiar with the problems which may arise, but which are actually simple to deal with. For example, skin scales may lodge between the rod and cylinder electrodes causing improper contact and hence, incorrect point detection. Therefore, before using the Punctoscope, you should push the cylinder back and clean the rod electrode. The batteries are weak or discharged if a constant buzzing signal is heard even when the probe electrode is not applied to the skin (i. e. without a closed circuit), or the device indicates no points at all. If you use your Punctoscope very often, you should replace the batteries every month.

The Treatment of the Correspondence Points

a) Needles

We use gold, molybdenum, silver, or steel needles to stimulate sensitive or electrically detected points. Here, we are again faced with the most frequently asked question in body acupuncture: What is the difference between the various metals, and when should which metal be used?

Although there is no definite scientific proof as yet as to the different effect of gold and silver needles, we can state that the action of precious metals is based on their own electrical potential. (According to *Wogralik,* gold has an electrical potential of + 0.285 and silver of only + 0.048 on the basis of the hydrogen electrode.) This potential is, however, increased by the contact potential after insertion of the needle into the tissue, resulting in an even greater potential difference.

In contrast to body acupuncture, incorrect selection of the metal of the needle manifests itself in ear acupuncture with immediate intensification of the peripheral complaints. This is the result of ear acupuncture's reflex action. The error can be corrected by using a different metal. As we have seen in the foregoing chapter, the Punctoscope can be of aid in the selection of the correct metal.

The patient's medical history, as well as the type of pain discovered during both the examination of the periphery and point detection on the ear, can also contribute to correct selection. Points which correspond with hypofunction require gold; points which reflect hyperfunction require silver. If the pain released by contact with the probe radiates over a large area of the ear, silver should be used. If it covers only a limited area, gold.
There are also several factors which suggest the use of a certain metal:

Gold: for pain
1. resulting from inflammations,
2. resulting from exhaustion,
3. resulting from hypofunction,
4. which increases when the specific function is called into action.

Silver: for pain
1. caused by hyperfunction,
2. which increases at rest and improves with movement,
3. caused by trauma.
When in doubt, we suggest using steel needles.

In recent years, we have, as a rule, been using stainless steel needles only at the Ludwig Boltzmann Acupuncture Institute. Experience has shown that, contrary to contradicting opinions, elimination of pain within a matter of seconds may also be achieved with stainless steel needles. Furthermore, stainless steel needles are much easier to sterilize. The use of precious metal needles necessitates separate sterilization of each metal, as ion migration causes gold needles to take on a silver, and silver needles a gold tinge, so that in no time, they can no longer be told apart. Stainless steel needles, in contrast, may be simply sterilized along with all body acupuncture needles of the same material.

The technique of needle insertion is very simple. The needle selected according to the above criteria is as a rule inserted into the skin perpendicularly to the surface down to the cartilage. The cartilage must not be injured; inserting the needle through it must be avoided. If the correct correspondence point is needled, the patient will grimace, jerk away, or exclaim, just as in manual point detection. The needle is rotated several times to increase the stimulus and achieve better results.

If electrical or vibratory stimulation is used, we suggest using a Chinese steel needle and advancing it subcutaneously parallel to the surface of the skin up to ½ cm to keep it from slipping out. It goes without saying that **every precaution must be taken to insure sterility.**

"Permanent" needles must be carefully checked as otherwise perichondritis may develop.

The period of time for which the needles remain in place varies; in general, about 15—20 minutes.

After the needles have been removed, you must watch for bleeding as this usually does not occur immediately, but only after several seconds have elapsed. Compression is usually sufficient to stop the bleeding.

b) Microcurrent

To make auricular therapy more agreeable or painless for children and anxious or extremely sensitive patients, *Nogier* had a special therapeutic device, the Therapunkteur P*) constructed according to his design. This device produces positive and negative, poled and alternating square-wave impulses with a capacity of 10 mA and a frequency of 1 Hz. This device can replace a gold needle with the positive pole, a silver needle with the negative pole, and a steel needle with alternating current.

---

*) Therapunkteur P. S. E. D. A. T. Co., France.

c) Combination Instrument for Point Detection and Electrical Stimulation

(The Punctoscope DT)

This instrument is a combination of the Punctoscope and the Therapunkteur P. With it, the points can not only be located according to reduced or increased skin resistance, but also electrically stimulated as well. The detector resembles that of the Punctoscope, also enabling evaluation of the point's resistance in comparison to that of the immediate surrounding area. The instrument has a special detector electrode to locate body points as well.

Procedure for use:

The Punctoscope DT is held by the patient, who switches it on by pressing the D-button (Diagnosis). The physician then adjusts the device to the individual sensibility of the side of the body to be examined as described on page 21, and then examines the areas he

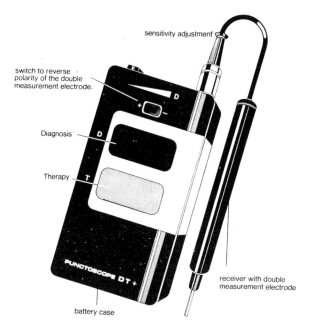

Fig. 5: Punctoscope DT*

---

*S. E. D. A. T. Co., France

25

has selected to find their maximum points. Has a point of therapeutic interest been found, the potentiometer being adjusted to low, the patient is then told to press the T-botton (Therapy). It goes without saying that the contact between detector electrode and skin remains unbroken.

Pressing the T-button starts electrical stimulation with an alternating current having an intensity of up to 60 μA and a frequency of about 1 Hz. This device is too new to allow me to make any conclusive statements based on experience obtained using it.

Laterality

Laterality is a significant problem inherent in auricular therapy. While mainly symmetrical points are used in body acupuncture (that is, almost every point lies on the left and on the right side of the body), in auricular therapy, you must find the "dominant" ear via which the therapy is to be performed.

In the majority of cases (about 90%) you will find active points on the ipsilateral ear, that is, on the same side as the disorder in the body. In about 2% of the cases, the corresponding points lie on the contralateral ear.

Various methods have been described for determining which auricle contains the main information. These methods are all quite complicated and time-consuming and are, as in the case of the auriculo-cardiac reflex (cutivascular reflex), dependent on the examiner's sensitivity and skill.

The following simple method has proven itself effective to me, and I have been using it successfully for many years:

First, I examine the corresponding projection areas on both ears with a probe or bellied bougie. The "dominant" ear, which contains the most information, is always more sensitive at this site than the other ear. The Punctoscope as well will always indicate a considerable difference of potential between the point and the skin surrounding it on the dominant ear.

Indications

Pain represents the main domain of auricular reflex therapy. Regardless of the location of the pain, or its cause, auricular therapy can always alleviate it or even make the patient free of pain. This, however, does not mean that failures never occur.

Pain is one of the main obstacles to rapid rehabilitation. Here, a quick response can be achieved via the reflex points. Auricular therapy is also very effective for postoperative or posttraumatic pain. It is also a good supplement to osteopathic manipulation or physical medicine, not only for diagnosis of the basic disorder, but also for testing the effectiveness of the manual treatment.

The various types of neuralgia (in any location), causalgia, headache, as well as pain of humoral or infectious origin, also fall under the heading of pain. Stomach, intestinal, and urogenital disturbances are the internal disorders which react best to auricular therapy. Allergic illnesses, especially allergic disorders of the nose and asthma, can also be favorably influenced. The range of therapeutic possibilities is very wide. However, regardless of the specific illness with which you are dealing, you must always keep the pathophysiological cause in mind. Only then will you be able to get to the root of the disorder. **Thus, standardized therapy programs are useless in auricular therapy.**

Contraindications

Absolute Contraindications

1. Pain which indicates the necessity of surgery (appendicitis, empyema of the gallbladder, etc.)

2. All degenerative and congenital disorders in which mainly the spinal cord is affected

3. Demyelinating diseases

4. Treatment of the thalamus point, the points on the intertragic notch, and the area corresponding with the inner genitals during pregnancy

5. Carcinomas; The pain they cause, however, may be treated.

Relative Contraindications

1. The period immediately following extreme physical and mental exertion

2. The hormonally active points during menstruation.

To the novice, the ear seems to be homogenous. Therefore, he must first become familiar with the anatomical characteristics, as the location of the reflex zones is dependent on the anatomic relief of the ear.

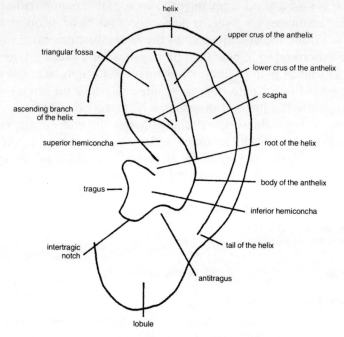

Fig. 6: The anatomy of the auricle

The Anatomy of the Auricle

On the outer ear, we differentiate a **surface plane** consisting of the auricle itself, the tragus, and the ascending branch of the helix and a **deep plane** formed by the concha.

1. The Surface Plane

The Helix

The helix represents the frame of the auricle like a border which mainly curves around the concave inner surface. 4 sections are differentiated:

a) The Root of the Helix, which actually belongs to the deep plane, lies in the concha which it divides into two parts.

b) The Ascending Branch of the Helix begins on the foremost portion of the root of the helix where it has a transverse indentation. The latter can be found with an instrument called the "stirrup"*). The O-point according to *Nogier* is also located here. The ascending branch curves forwards on the top. Its beginning portion is narrow, then it widens and flattens forming a more or less triangular surface. Its dorsal side hangs over the frontal portion of the superior hemiconcha and the frontal portion of the lower crus of the anthelix.

Two areas are noteworthy:
1. The neural centers of the genitals project to the outer surface.
2. The internal genitals project to the inner surface; the projection of the kidneys lies above them.

c) The Body of the Helix
which forms the peripheral frame of the auricle

d) The Tail of the Helix
which forms the terminal, cartilaginous part of the frame of the ear and ends on the fleshy portion of the earlobe.
There is another noteworthy fold in the auricle:

The Anthelix

The anthelix represents the border between the auricle and the concha and arises from 2 roots on the anterior, upper portion of the auricle which unite to form its body.

a) The lower crus
begins beneath the ascending branch of the helix. It is narrow and angular, and protrudes over the uppermost portion of the superior hemiconcha (projection of the coccyx, and the sacral and lumbar vertebrae).

---

*) The "stirrup" is a thick u-shaped wire. A fine wire is soldered across the two open ends. This instrument is not only helpful in locating the O-point, but also in locating the projections of the individual vertebrae on the anthelix.

b) The upper crus
is wider and more protrusive. It begins in the anterior quarter of
the upper portion of the auricle.

c) The body of the anthelix
The two crura unite to form the body of the anthelix. The thoracic
and cervical vertebrae project onto it. It ends above **the antitragus,**
a triangular protrusion overlapping the inferior hemiconcha. The
anthelix and the antitragus are separated from each other by the
distinct indentation of the **posterior antitragal groove** (projection
of the atlanto-occipital joint).

There are also two other indentations in the auricle:

a) Before they unite, the crura of the anthelix form the borders
of a triangular indentation, the triangular or navicular fossa (projection of the lower extremities).

b) A boat-shaped depression is found between the body of the
helix and the upper crus of the anthelix. This is called the **scapha,**
or the **groove of the helix.** The greatest portion of its surface represents the projection of the upper extremities. The lower portion
corresponds with the neck. The maxilla and mandible lie on the
transition area from the scapha to the lobe of the ear.

Below the ascending branch of the helix, we find triangular-
shaped cartilage, the **tragus,** which protrudes over the external auditory meatus. The tragus and antitragus are separated by a deep
notch, the **intertragic notch.**

2. The Deep Plane

The Concha

The anthelix forms the upper and dorsal border of the concha;
the antitragus forms the dorsal lower border. The anterior border
is formed by the opening of the external auditory meatus and the
tragus. The intertragic notch, which lies between the tragus and antitragus, represents the lower border.

The concha is divided into sections by the root of the helix: the
superior hemiconcha, to which the abdominal viscera project, and
the **inferior hemiconcha.**

The **inferior hemiconcha** consists of two planes:
a) a vertical plane to which the thoracic organs project, and
b) a horizontal plane on the level of the intertragic notch. This is also called the foot of the concha. Portions of the projection of the diencephalon (hypothalamus and hypophysis) are found here.

The Innervation of the Auricle

The innervation represents the theoretical foundation of reflex therapy via the ear. The immediate reactions occurring in the majority of cases which are comparable to the "Sekundenphänomen" (disappearance of pain within a matter of seconds) show that reflex mechanisms must play a role. Indeed, the general opinion is that only when a positive effect, i. e. disappearance of pain, appears immediately after insertion of the needles, have the correct points been chosen.

In my opinion, research on the embryogenesis and, therewith, the innervation of the auricle, has not yet been completed. *Bossy,*

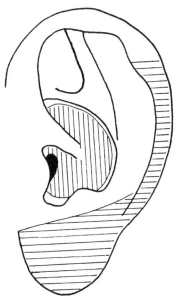

Fig. 7: The innervation of the auricle ▦= Auricular ramus of the vagus ◻= auriculotemporal nerve (N. V.) ≡ = great auricular nerve (cervical plexus)

31

Nogier, Bourdiol, and many other co-workers are working on research in this field of anatomy. I believe that clarification of the neuroanatomical relationships in the ear will be the key to the discovery of the mechanism elicited by stimulation of the auricle.

All leading anatomists are of the opinion that the auricle is innervated by three nerves: the vagus nerve, the cervical plexus, and the trigeminal nerve.

1. The Auricular Ramus of the Vagus Nerve

represents a sensitive branch of the innervation area of the vagus in the head. It supplies the entire concha, but does not conform to its normal borders. Hence, it does not supply the anthelix, the antitragus, or the anterior upper angle of the superior hemiconcha.

2. The Great Auricular Nerve

from the cervical plexus innervates the dorsal middle portion of the helix and the lobule below the subantitragic fold.

According to Nogier, the lobule is innervated by the glossopharyngeal nerve. This hypothesis is based on the embryological fact that the 9th cranial nerve is the nerve of the third branchial arch and lies between the 5th nerve (first branchial arch), the 7th nerve (second branchial arch), and the 10th nerve (fourth branchial arch), all of which are represented in the auricle. However, even the newest anatomy books contain no reference thereto.

3. The Auriculotemporal Branch

of the trigeminal nerve supplies the rest of the auricle, hence, the ascending branch of the helix, the anterior portion of the helix up to the innervation border of the cervical plexus, the triangular fossa, scapha, anthelix, antitragus, and the margin of the concha which is not innervated by the vagus.

Via this abundant innervation, the auricle has important connections to the cerebrospinal system. These again are significantly increased by the connections to the autonomic nervous system. However, just this very same vegetative supply in the auricle has been much less the subject of exact investigation than has been the sensitive, although it is, in my opinion, of much greater significance in auricular therapy. Of the numerous publications which have appeared in the past years on the subject of auricular reflex therapy, that of *Kwirtschischvile* (cited in "Akupunktur, Theorie und Praxis" 1/1974) stands out in particular:

"After having applied terpentine to the musculature of rabbits' extremities, the changes in skin resistance at the correspondence zones of the auricle were registered. Aside from the known reduction of skin resistance on 'active' points, other functional and morphological changes were observed in the sense of transudation, hyperemia, and scabbing. Following extirpation of the superior cervical ganglia, there was no change in the auricle, the same experimental model having been used. In contrast, severing the somatic nerves did not hinder reaction in the projection zone. The observed manifestations on the projection zones may therefore be caused by local changes in vessels and glands, these being innervated via the sympathetic nerve system."

We have concluded our general observations on the auricle and now turn to the specific reflex cartography.

The Reflex Cartography of the Auricle

Bones, Muscles and Joints

The Projection of the Spinal Column

The spinal column projects to the foremost portion of the lower crus and body of the anthelix. The projection extends from the posterior antitragal groove (projection of the atlas) to the foremost portion of the lower crus of the anthelix, which is covered by the ascending branch of the helix (projection of the coccyx).

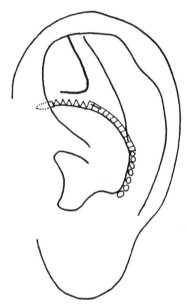

Fig. 8: The projection of the spinal column (after *Nogier*) O = cervical vertebrae □ = thoracic vertebrae △ = lumbar vertebrae ⊙ = sacrum and coccyx

---

For a better three-dimensional projection in studying the points I have developed a plastic ear model in which the most important points of the ear acupuncture are marked. One can obtain it through Karl F. Haug Publishers, Heidelberg.

The reflex zones of the individual sections of the spinal column can be precisely determined. The borders between the cervical and thoracic vertebrae, as well as between the thoracic and lumbar vertebrae are represented by transverse depressions on the margin of the anthelix.

These notches or depressions, which are barely visible, can be easily located with the instrument designed by *Nogier*, the "stirrup". If you move this instrument over the free margin of the anthelix using somewhat more pressure, you will automatically stop at these depressions and thus be able to differentiate the individual sections of the spinal column. Even careful inspection is sufficient for separating or differentiating the individual sections because their directions vary. Hence, you can easily see that the radius of the curvature of the individual spinal sections on the anthelix varies. The radius of the projection of the cervical vertebrae is significantly smaller than that of the thoracic vertebrae.

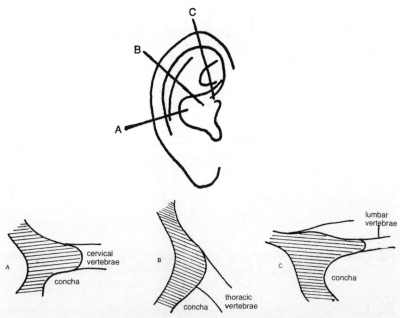

Fig. 9: Cross section through the anthelix on the level of the A) cervical vertebrae, B) thoracic vertebrae, and C) lumbar vertebrae (modified according to *Nogier*)

The cross section of the relief of the anthelix also shows a distinct variation in each section. In conformity with *Nogier's* basic concept that the auricle corresponds with a fetus in its normal term position in the uterus, i.e. upside down, the cervical vertebrae are found in the lower portion and the lumbar vertebrae in the uppermost portion of the anthelix.

1. The Cervical Vertebrae

The cervical vertebrae project to the lowest portion of the body of the anthelix and are almost vertical. Here, the cross section shows a rather small radius. The projection begins above the antitragus congruous with the posterior antitragal groove. The atlanto-occipital joint projects to this depression.

The 3rd cervical vertebra projects to the point of intersection of the anthelix with an imaginary line representing the continuation of the root of the helix.

The upper border of this portion is the cervicothoracic depression under which the **7th cervical vertebra is found.**

2. The Thoracic Vertebrae

Above the cervicothoracic depression, the radius of curvature becomes distinctly larger. Simultaneously, the cross section of the relief shows a wider curve. The projection of the thoracic vertebrae extends to the next large depression, the thoracolumbar depression, which lies across from the tip of the triangular fossa.

3. The Lumbar Vertebrae

This zone projects to the lower crus of the anthelix. Above the thoracolumbar depression, the free margin of the anthelix bends sharply forwards, then becoming practically horizontal. At the same time, the edge of the margin becomes quite sharp.

The termination of the lumbar region is marked by another, easily located depression. This corresponds with the lumbosacral articulation at the level of the point of intersection with the margin of the ascending branch of the helix.

4. The Sacrum and Coccyx

This projection is equally divided between the sacrum and coccyx on the anterior portion of the lower crus of the anthelix, and is completely covered by the ascending branch of the helix. You must bend the latter back in order to closely inspect this zone.

The study group in Lyon was able to establish even more exact locations in the region of the spinal column reflex zones: The projection of the homolateral half of the vertebral body with its transverse process lies on the tip of the free margin of the anthelix, while the intervertebral disk is located in that part of the anthelix adjoining the above location oriented towards the concha.

If you precisely differentiate the individual sections of the spinal column, you will be able to make an exact diagnosis of the disturbed vertebra with a probe or the Punctoscope by correctly dividing the located section (cervical vertebrae: 7 parts, thoracic vertebrae: 12, lumbar vertebrae: 5). The points which are sensitive to pressure, or can be electrically located, correspond with the vertebral segment which may be disturbed.

Post-traumatic conditions, such as fractures or fissures of vertebrae, can also be established in this manner. However, you must always bear in mind that these diagnostic or therapeutic methods can only act on the corresponding vertebra. Repositioning is impossible (caution: transverse lesions). However, this can take place via "spontaneous realignment" when pain has been eliminated.

The Paravertebral Projection

As I have mentioned above, the projections of the vertebral bodies lie on the protruding part of the anthelix. Two other noteworthy locations are found parallel to this:

1. The reflex area of the paravertebral ligaments and muscles is found behind the edge of the body of the anthelix and the lower crus of the anthelix, hence, towards the scapha and triangular fossa. The surface vessels and nerves of the neck are also found in the region of the cervical vertebrae. Via the corresponding level of this area, pain which is caused by ligaments or muscle contraction (e. g. lumbago) can be diagnosed and treated.

When dealing with cases of cervicobrachial neuralgia, you will have to carefully examine points of this zone in the region of the cervical vertebrae. Also headaches which are caused by paravertebral muscular rigidity and which radiate from the neck to the forehead, are treated via this area.

2. The projection of the paravertebral sympathetic system (paravertebral ganglia) lies parallel to the projection of the spinal column in the depression formed by the transition from anthelix to concha.

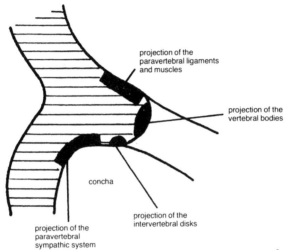

projection of the
paravertebral ligaments
and muscles

projection of the
vertebral bodies

concha

projection of the
intervertebral disks

projection of the
paravertebral
sympathic system

Fig. 10: Cross section through the anthelix with the projections of the vertebral bodies, intervertebral disks, and the paravertebral sympathetic system

It includes the area of the concha which is not innervated by the auricular ramus of the vagus nerve. Via this region, neurovegetative disturbances, such as those associated with fused vertebrae or whiplash injuries, or in cervical migraine, can be influenced.

This zone will be discussed later in the section on the projection of the vegetative (autonomic) nervous system.

The Projection of the Upper Extremities

This reflex area comprises the entire area between the upper crus of the anthelix and the helix, and fills the entire scapha or groove of the helix.

If we observe the disproportionately large projection of the upper extremity on the ear, we see for the first time a marked congruence with the disproportionately large sensory and motor cortical areas of the hand. The projection areas on the cerebral cortex also show a division in which the corresponding sections of the body are cortically represented.

The size of the area does not reflect the bulk of the muscle or the size of a sensory field, but rather the number of motor units or the number of receptors. Hence, the size of the projection corresponds with the extent of dexterity with which the specific part of the body is able to perform precise voluntary movements. The more specific movements a muscle is able to make, the larger is its cortical area.

Thus, the **thumb** with its manifold movement possibilities comprises a particularly large area in the cerebral cortex as well as in its projection on the ear. On the ear, its region extends parallel to the upper crus of the anthelix, from the superior fold of the helix (tip of the thumb) to the level of the angle of the triangular fossa (ball of the thumb or wrist).

The other fingers lie dorsal to the thumb whereby the fingertips lie in the upper part of the scapha covered by the folded down edge of the helix.

The wrist is found at the level of the union of the crura of the anthelix.

The elbow lies on the level of the lower crus of the anthelix.

The shoulder girdle lies on the level of the 7th cervical and 1st thoracic vertebrae.

The projection of **the lower arm** is found between the elbow and wrist. The radius comprises the anterior portion, and the ulna the posterior portion.

The Projection of the Lower Extremities

The triangular fossa represents the reflex location of the lower extremities. Hence, **the big toe** is found in the posterior upper part of the fossa approaching the upper crus of the anthelix, exactly across from the projection of the thumb. The other toes adjoin it so that **the small (fifth) toe** lies under the ascending branch of the helix in the anterior portion of the triangular fossa.

The ankle and heel lie in the anterior lower fourth of the fossa. The heel is located close to the anthelix on the level of the sacrum. In order to locate this, you must bend back the ascending branch of the helix as the point lies exactly beneath it.

The ankle is found above and somewhat behind the heel. The internal malleolus lies somewhat lower on the level of the 5th lum-

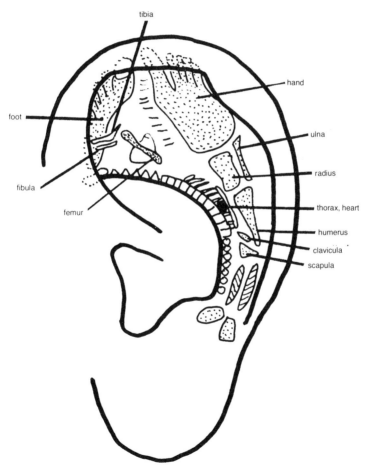

Fig. 11: Schematic projection of the extremities

41

bar vertebra; the external malleolus higher, on the level of the projection of the sacrum.

The joint of the knee is the easiest to locate. It projects to the deepest point of the fossa.

You can also use the "knee point" as an orientation point for locating the projections of the tibia, fibula, and femur. In relation to the knee point, the zone of the **tibia** is situated anteriorly and above, the **fibula** anteriorly and below, and the **femur** posteriorly and below.

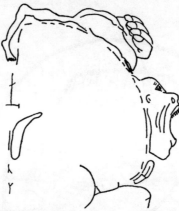

Fig. 12: Somatotopic projection fields on the cerebral cortex (after *Penfield* and *Rasmussen,* 1950)

The hip joint comprises the tip of the fossa. The projection of the gluteal muscles lies somewhat in front of it, above the lower crus of the anthelix.

The zone corresponding with the **sciatic nerve** is found halfway between the gluteal muscles and the heel.

Some of the projection zones of the lower extremities presented in currently available Chinese ear charts differ considerably from those after *Nogier.* For example, the Chinese projection of the heel-bone is found in the region of the upper crus of the anthelix, while *Nogier* has placed it in the triangular fossa.

This prompted *Kiszel* of Vienna's General Emergency Hospital, to carry out comparative investigations of cases having heel-bone and ankle joint fractures, as these zones differ most: Sixteen patients having a total of 20 heel-bone fractures were investigated. Of these, 9 were set and fixed with drill wire. Three patients had bilateral heel-bone fractures; one patient had a fracture of the left heel-bone and a dislocation fracture of the right ankle; and two patients had a compression fracture at the distal end of the tibia on the other leg, aside from heel-bone fractures.

Both projections were examined on both ears with the Punctoscope.

These investigations clearly show that *Nogier's* projection location is correct.

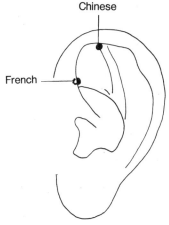

Fig. 13: Chinese and French projections of the heel-bone

The Projection of the Thoracic Skeletal Structure

This chapter shall only deal with the projections of the bones, muscles, and ligaments of the thorax. The thoracic organs, with the exception of the heart, lie in the inferior hemiconcha.

The **thorax,** with the sternum and ribs, occupies the middle third of the anthelix. The ribs' projections lie behind the corresponding thoracic vertebrae. The sternum lies somewhat farther dorsal.

In relation to the projection of the thoracic vertebrae, this zone extends from the 2nd to the 8th thoracic vertebra. In women who complain of pain in the region of the pectoral muscle, points will always manifest themselves in this zone.

Patient's age	Injury and degree of severity (I–VI)		Sensitivity in the auricle		Projection French School		Chinese School		Intensity on the Puncto-scope-scale	Point in time after accident at which examination took place
	l	r	l	r	l	r	l	r		
24 a	heel-bone fracture VI, op.	disloc fracture of the ankle	+	+	+	+			4	after 12 weeks
40 a		heel-bone fracture VI, op	(+)			+ scale formation			5	after 14 weeks
25 a	heel-bone fracture VI, op.	heel-bone fracture II			+	+			5	after 14 weeks
55 a		heel-bone fracture V				+		+	6	after 12 weeks
36 a	heel-bone fracture V, op.	heel-bone fracture II			+	+	+		4	after 12 weeks
35 a	heel-bone fracture V, op.	dist. compound fracture of the tibia		+	+	heel + ankle + knee +			4	after 14 weeks
29 a	heel-bone fracture IV	heel-bone fracture II	+	+	+	+			5	after 2 hours

Age	Diagnosis				Punctoscope	Grade	Time
27 a	heel-bone fracture V and dist. fracture of the tibia *(heel-bone fracture V)*	+		+	+ (intensity 6 on the Punctoscope)	4	after 4 months
19 a	heel-bone fracture V, op.	+	+	+	+ (intensity 6 on the Punctoscope)	4	after 12 weeks
42 a	heel-bone fracture IV	+		+		4	after 5 months
37 a	heel-bone fracture V, op.	+		+		4	after 12 weeks
65 a	heel-bone fracture V	+		+		5	after 10 weeks
69 a	heel-bone fracture V	+		+		5	after 8 weeks
34 a	heel-bone fracture V, op.	+	+	+	heel + / knee +	5	after 14 weeks
67 a	heel-bone fracture V			±		5	after 10 weeks
36 a	heel-bone fracture V, op.		+			5	after 12 weeks

Tab. 1

The shoulder blade lies somewhat in front of and below the described shoulder area on the body of the anthelix behind the 6th cervical to 2nd thoracic vertebra.

Nogier also locates the **heart** in this projection zone. In contrast to his original concept, in which he located the heart in the inferior hemiconcha at the level of the posterior antitragal groove, the projection is now located at the level of the ribs corresponding to the 4th and 5th thoracic vertebrae.

Nogier arrived at the latter location through contemplation of developmental anatomy according to which the organs and the skeletal system, which are of mesodermic genesis, project exclusively to that area of the ear innervated by the trigeminal nerve. Since the heart also arises from the mesodermic layer, its projection must also be located in the area innervated by the 5th cranial nerve. Therefore, its original location in the concha (which is of endodermal origin) is no longer valid.

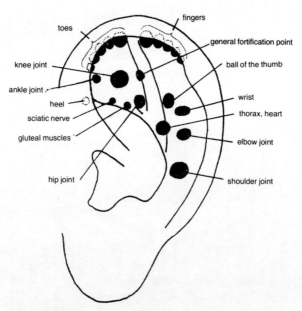

Fig. 14: Specific zones of the upper and lower extremities

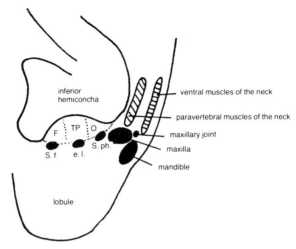

Fig. 15: Zones of the cranial bones, sinuses, maxilla, mandible, and muscles of the neck

S. f.	= frontal sinus	F	= frontal region
e. l.	= ethmoidal labyrinth	TP	= temporoparietal region
S. ph.	= sphenoidal sinus	O	= occipital region

Numerous studies on angina pectoris patients, all of whom demonstrate points which are sensitive to pressure in this zone, show that this, newer localization of the projection is correct.

The Projection of the Neck

The reflex zones of this region lie in the isthmus of the auricle in the region of the 3rd—6th cervical vertebra. The muscles of the neck are of primary interest here. The ventral portions, in particular the **sternocleidomastoid muscle,** lie in the dorsal portion of the isthmus towards the anterior edge of the root of the helix. The paravertebral muscles (scalenus, rhomboid, trapezius muscles) are situated in the anterior portion of the isthmus, oriented towards the body of the anthelix. Muscular tension in the region of the neck, including the area of the shoulder blade, can be influenced via this zone. Spastic torticollis is an exception as it is an extrapyramidal hyperkinetic disorder with lesions in the region of the striatum. The same applies to congenital torticollis caused by scar tissue.

47

The Projection of the Skull

The reflex area of the cranial bones is the antitragus. The antitragus is a triangular protrusion which partly overhangs the inferior hemiconcha, forming its dorsal, lower border. Looking cranially, the antitragus is separated from the anthelix by the posterior antitragal groove; frontally the intertragic notch separates it from the tragus; downwards towards the earlobe, it is bordered by the supralobular crease.

The antitragus consists of two planes: an inner plane which faces the concha, and an outer plane. Let us examine the latter.

The outer plane of the antitragus represents the projection area of the bony portion of the cranium as well as the corresponding cerebral formation and its vessels.

The projection of the **frontal bone** and **frontal lobe** is found in the anterior third of this plane. The **temporal** and **parietal** bones and the **temporal** and **parietal lobes** lie in the middle third. The projection of the **occipital bone** and **occipital lobe** is found in the dorsal third. These zones must be examined and treated particularly when the patient complains of headache in the corresponding regions.

The reflex zones of the **sinuses** lie on a narrow margin on the outer, lower border of the antitragus just in front of the transition area to the lobule in the region of the supralobular crease.

The frontal sinus lies below the reflex location of the frontal bone. Beneath it, approximately on the level of the upper third of the lobule, lies an area which may be used for all types of disorders of smell and anosmia.

The ethmoid bone (ethmoid cells) lies beneath the parietal bone. **The sphenoid bone** lies beneath the occipital bone. All sinus problems, be they inflammatory or painful, can be influenced via these locations.

The reflex zone of the **mandible** lies in the dorsal section of the end of the scapha (cartilagenous portion) below the antitragus.

The tempero-mandibular joint is represented beneath the posterior antitragal groove on the border between scapha and lobule.

The projection of the **maxilla** is found in the anterior section of the scapha behind and below the location of the occipital bone.

Pain caused by trigeminal neuralgia, sinusitis, pulpitis, and pain in the region of the tempero-mandibular joints is treated via this zone.

That concludes the discussion of the somatic projections. These are exactly determined areas within which the maximum points for reflex therapy of functional or painful disorders of exactly definable anatomic locations may be addressed.

In reading the next chapter on the projection zones of the nervous system, it must be kept in mind that the given areas have been determined only upon the evidence of therapeutic results in common syndromes.

The Nervous System

General Outline

1. The Projection of the Central Nervous System

The description of the individual areas of the CNS corresponds with the hierarchical structure of the brain.

A) The projection of the telencephalon (or cerebrum) with its four large lobes (frontal lobe, temporoparietal, occipital) and the rhinencephalon with the limbic cortex are found on the outer plane of the antitragus and the entire lobule adjoining it.

The cerebral convolutions project to the antitragus while the lobule reflects the zones of simple mental integration.

B) The projection of the diencephalon lies on the inner surface of the antitragus and on the foot of the concha (horizontal portion of the inferior hemiconcha). Of its four main nuclei, the thalamus, epithalamus, metathalamus, and hypothalamus, we are mainly interested in the thalamus and hypothalamus.

Because of their anatomical proximity and physiological correlation with the hypophysis, their projections shall be discussed in that section.

C) The projection of the mesencephalon (or midbrain) lies below the external auditory meatus, separated however from the projection of the diencephalon.

D) The projection of the sensory and motor roots of the spinal cord is found on the helix.

The Specific Sections

A) The Projection of the Telencephalon (Cerebrum)

a) The Zone of the Frontal Lobe: This zone lies in the anterior region of the earlobe. Here, the **prefrontal cortex** is of particular interest. It comprises the foremost part of this area.

The intertragic notch forms the upper boundary of this zone. From there, the boundary travels downwards to just in front of the lowest edge of the lobule. Hence, an approximately triangular area is traced.

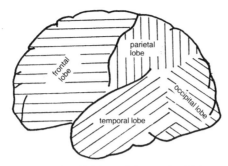

Fig. 16: The division of the cerebral lobes

This zone is especially effective for emotional disorders and poor concentration. This zone must also be thoroughly examined in cases of chronic pain or psychosomatic pain, and the points discovered must be included in the therapy program. The effect of these points is similar to that of tranquilizers.

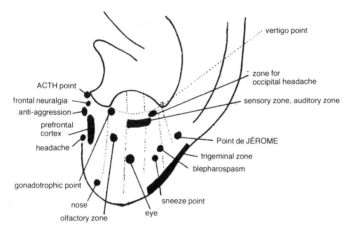

Fig. 17: The projection of the telencephalon

One zone is particularly noteworthy:

The Anti-Aggression Zone

This zone lies below the ACTH point near the junction of the earlobe and cheek just about on the point of intersection of two

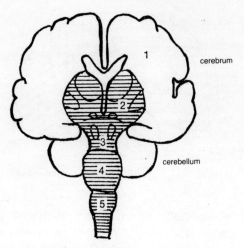

Fig. 18: Comparison of the cerebrum and the brain stem (hatched). 1 = telencephalon, 2 = diencephalon, 3 = mesencephalon, 4 = metencephalon, 5 = myelencephalon.

imaginary lines: a horizontal line through the angle helix — lobule and a vertical line through the foremost boundary of the intertragic notch. This reflex zone may be used for all forms of aggression. *Nogier* even uses it on married couples who no longer get along or for behavior problems in adolescents. This zone must always be included in the **therapy of addiction** be it nicotine, narcotic, drug addiction, or obesity. It serves to inhibit the neurotic withdrawal symptoms which usually include irritability and aggressiveness.

In practice, this location varies in size depending on the intensity of the dominating emotion. Hence, a simple aggressive thought will express itself in a small, very limited point, while a pronounced hatred will cover a larger area.

If the aggression is even greater, for example, if an act of violence is being planned, an area on the medial surface of the earlobe corresponding to the above-described area can be detected. According to experience, this area is found on the right earlobe in right-handed persons and on the left earlobe in left-handed persons (see also Fig. 34).

This zone is acupunctured with a silver needle for all of the above-described indications. Several needles are used if the area is larger (possibly cribriform needling).

A gold needle is inserted into this point for **hypothyroidism** to achieve appropriate mentally activating reactions and for **anorexia.**

b) The Zone of the Limbic Cortex (Rhinencephalon): The lower frontal regions of the cerebral cortex and those located around the brain stem, which used to be called the rhinencephalon, do not only have an olfactory function. The greater part is responsible for emotional reactions and complex neuro-endocrine regulatory functions.

Therefore, the term limbic cortex or limbic system is more appropriate. Phylogenetically speaking, it is the oldest part of the cerebral cortex. Inner cortical sections, for example, the amygdaloid nucleus, also belong to these cortical parts.

That both systems are closely connected can be clearly seen on the projection zone on the lobule in which the points corresponding with the sexual sphere can be found next to olfactory points.

The former correspond with the amygdaloid nucleus. This zone is found behind the prefrontal zone on the lobule in a narrow margin which also includes the foremost third of the antitragus. Five noteworthy points are found in this area:

1. The projection of the frontal sinus lies on the border between the antitragus and the lobule. It manifests itself in cases of neuralgia from sinusitis in the frontal region.

2. Vasomotor frontal headache can be alleviated with points in the anterior third of the antitragus.

3. The olfactory zone's location is found in the middle of the zone margin on the level of the anterior attachment of the earlobe. It must be carefully examined in cases of disorders of smell or anosmia.

4. The nasal zone lies in the lower region of this area. It corresponds to the spot one pinches with the fingertips during sneezing attacks. It is used for all nasal disorders, especially for allergic conditions.

The connection of the limbic zone to the sexual sphere exists through the immediate proximity of its upper portion to the gonadotrophic point. The latter lies on the junction of the anterior attachment of the antitragus and the intertragic notch.

c) The Zone of the Temporal Lobe adjoins the limbic zone dorsally and comprises almost the upper half of the lobule in the extension of the middle third of the antitragus.

In the region of the antitragus, it represents the temporoparietal cortical portion. The region lying on the earlobe corresponds with the transverse temporal gyri (Heschl's gyrus) mainly connected with the sense of hearing.

A transverse zone, **the sensory zone** according to *Nogier,* is found on the lobule somewhat below the middle third of the antitragus. It can be used for the treatment of certain types of tinnitus (silver needle).

Treatment of this zone with a gold needle can also influence certain types of hearing impairment. This zone is also supposed to influence the **memory**.

The **projection of the eye** lies on the center point of the earlobe (optic impressions are intensified: one "sees better" when the point is stimulated with a gold needle).

d) The Zone of the Occipital Lobe projects to the area adjoining the temporal zone in a margin which widens towards the lower edge of the lobule. It extends upwards to the dorsal third of the antitragus. On its border to the lobule a zone is found which has a favorable influence on **headache** radiating from the occiput to the forehead. The immediate proximity of the projection of the vertebral artery and the atlanto-occipital articulation also confirms the effectiveness of this area for the treatment of vertigo in connection with **cervical syndrome.**

e) The Zone of the Cerebellum: Originally, this zone was considered to be located in front of the posterior antitragal groove extending to the dorsal upper portion of the horizontal plane of the inferior hemiconcha. According to more recent studies by *Nogier,* it lies on the medial surface of the auricle (see Fig. 38).

The positive results achieved by stimulating the projections of sensory functions on the lobule, such as sight, hearing, and sense of smell, are to be considered as activation of mental functions only, and do not, therefore, provide any experimental correlate.

Patients say that they feel their sight has improved, they hear more clearly, etc., allowing the assumption that the respective degree of activity of the mental function (attention) is increased.

The Zone of the Trigeminal Nerve

Although this zone does not actually belong to this section, I still wish to discuss it here. It lies on the lower edge of the earlobe and extends from the helix-lobule angle forwards to approximately the level of the dorsal third of the antitragus. It must be examined extremely carefully in cases of pain in the innervation area of the trigeminal nerve (see also the chapter "The Projection of the Parasympathetic System").

The Point de Jérome is found above the trigeminal zone on the transition of the tail of the helix to the lobule. This point is able to inhibit sexual drives. It was named after Hieronimus *Bosch,* who depicted a devil with a spear through exactly this point on a disproportionately large ear in his triptych "The Garden of Delights". In general, it is a tension-relieving point, and is also used in the treatment of insomnia.

B) The Projection of the Diencephalon

The most important nuclear regions of the diencephalon located around the central lacuna of the third ventricle are the **thalamus** and **hypothalamus.**

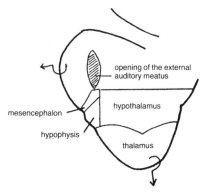

opening of the external auditory meatus

mesencephalon

hypothalamus

hypophysis

thalamus

Fig. 19: Overall view of the projection of the diencephalon and mesencephalon in the region of the horizontal plane of the inferior hemiconcha (foot of the concha). (The tragus bent forwards, the antitragus backwards)

The hypophysis shall also be discussed in this chapter, as the neurohypophysis (posterior lobe of the pituitary gland) extends from the base of the 3rd ventricle, and topographical physiological connections also exist.

a) The Projection of the Thalamus

Anatomically, the thalamus is the last switching location of all pathways ascending to the telencephalon with the exception of the olfactory tract. It represents a pre-cerebrum or "gate to the consciousness" so to speak, the last location from which the cerebral cortex derives sensory stimuli (tactile, visual, and auditory). It is also said to be an independent integration center in which the stimuli conducted from the sensory organs are supplemented by the simple sensations and affects, all of which is then passed on to the cerebral cortex.

On the auricle, the close connection between the thalamus and the cerebrum is also revealed, the projection zone of the former being on the inner surface of the antitragus, and that of the latter on the outer surface.

Several extremely important points are found in the thalamus zone on the inner surface of the antitragus. One stands out in particular:

The Thalamus Point

This point lies in the middle of the base of the antitragus (concha-side) on the border to the concha. It is easy to find if you pull the antitragus downwards and, using the fold thus formed as a guideline, proceed downwards towards the concha. At the end of the fold you will find a small groove in which this point lies.

Indications:

1. This point is able to alleviate or even eliminate all unilateral, usually homolateral, pain in the body (corresponds with the nucleus ventrocaudalis).

2. It is effective to a certain degree in the treatment of tics.

3. Interestingly, systolic blood pressure can be regulated via this point. Here, the metal of the needle used plays a very important role.

If the thalamus point is acupunctured with a gold needle, the blood pressure is lowered. Stimulation with a silver needle raises the blood pressure level. Pregnancy is a **contraindication** for acupuncture of this point.

The Tic Line

Nogier gave this name to the entire fold formed when the antitragus is folded down, from the tip of the antitragus to the thalamus point because several points can be found on it in cases with hyperkinetic disturbances or uncontrolled movements. These points are able to influence these disorders (corresponding to the physiological action of the anterolateral ventral thalamic nuclei).

The Sleep Point

This point lies on the anteriormost part of the inner surface of the antitragus symmetrical to the genital point which lies on the outer surface (e. g. hypophysis). It corresponds to the medial thalamic nucleus and is used for all sleep disorders.

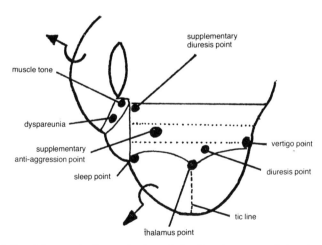

Fig. 20: Special zones in the projection of the di and mesencephalon (tragus bent forwards, antitragus outwards)

The Vertigo Point

This point lies on the dorsal, lower border of the inner surface of the antitragus to the concha. It corresponds to the projection of the carotid plexus and should be examined in cases of vertigo of vascular cause.

b) The Projection of the Hypothalamus

Aside from its regulating influence on the anterior and posterior lobe function of the hypophysis, the hypothalamus is also closely connected with autonomic functions.

We shall discuss the latter in this section.

The hypothalamus was once called "the main ganglion of the autonomic nervous system." Indeed, stimulation of the hypothalamus produces numerous autonomic effects. However, the autonomic effects released via the hypothalamus are frequently only the accompanying symptoms of more complex phenomena (i. e. anger and other emotions). However, there is very little evidence of the hypothalamus being a regulator of visceral functions.

Its reflex region on the ear comprises a trapezoid area in the horizontal part of the inferior hemiconcha. Looking inwards, it is bordered by an imaginary line running from below the opening of the external auditory meatus to the inner slope of the posterior antitragal groove. The base of the antitragus constitutes the outer border. Anteriorly, it adjoins the projection of the hypophysis.

Although physiologically-speaking, the hypothalamus demonstrates only sympathetic effects and no parasympathetic center has yet been found, there is one function set off by auricular stimulation which corresponds with a parasympathetic effect: contraction of the bladder.

In fact, there is a reflex area which lies somewhat towards the concha and behind the thalamus point which has a distinct influence on diuresis: **the diuresis point.** When it is stimulated, the bladder voids.

To obtain a better overall view of the location of the points of the hypothalamic region, it is divided into 3 strips of equal size which lie parallel to the base of the antitragus. The diuresis point is found in the outermost strip.

In cases of aggression, an extremely pressure-sensitive point is found in the middle region in front of the thalamus point. This is **the supplementary anti-aggression point** which corresponds anatomically to the lateral hypothalamic region.

Another diuresis point lies on the anterior border of the posterior strip near the projection of the hypophysis (posterior lobe of the pituitary gland). Stimulation of this point produces a distinct effect on certain types of edema (stimulation of the osmoreceptors in the anterior hypothalamus?).

Even more points seem to be hidden in this extremely interesting zone of the hypothalamus. They will only be found through further intensive research. I am thinking here of points which could aid in influencing appetite or thirst.

The hypothalamus, being the center of all processes of the vegetative system, is so closely related to the hypophysis which is responsible for hormonal regulation, that we can generally speak of a diencephalic-hypophyseal system.

This is also demonstrated on the ear by the close proximity of the two systems.

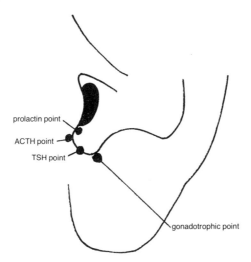

Fig. 21: Intertragic notch with hypophyseal glandular regulation points (tragus bent forwards, antitragus outwards)

c) The Projection of the Hypophysis

The hypophysis is a bean-shaped body which hangs as an appendage from the diencephalon. It consists of the adenohypophysis (anterior lobe) and the neurohypophysis (posterior lobe).

The entire hypophysis projects to an area which extends from the intertragic notch to the lower edge of the external auditory meatus.

Of the two portions, the projection of the anterior lobe on the auricle is of the most interest to us. The anterior lobe with its glandular regulation points projects to the narrow region of the intertragic notch. The following points are found there:

1. The Gonadotrophic Point

Corresponding to the gonadotrophic pituitary hormone, it lies on the point of intersection of the anterior outer edge of the antitragus with the intertragic notch, that is, about 1 mm below the dorsal border of the notch. Via this point, both the male and female genital function can be influenced; dysmenorrhea, meno and metrorrhagia, climacteric complaints in women.

Via this point one can also act indirectly on joints and skin if the complaints are connected with the menstrual cycle or first appear during menopause.

Note: A gold needle is used for menorrhagia or delayed menses. A silver needle is used for metrorrhagia and premature menstrual bleeding.

2. The ACTH Point

The projection is found in the foremost part of the intertragic notch on its border to the tragus. It lies somewhat beyond the edge, about 1 mm towards the cheek, hence, symmetrical to the genital point.

It is used in cases of mental and physical exhaustion, and must be considered for the treatment of painful disorders of the joints and spondylopathy.

3. The TSH Point (thyrotrophic hormone)

This point lies exactly in the axis of the intertragic canal, 1 mm inwards from its free edge.

This point has a favorable effect on the thyroid for both hypofunction and hyperfunction. Thus, it is not only able to influence asthenic conditions which include hypothyroid complaints (i.e. sensation of coldness), but also hyperactivity, irritability, and vascular instability such as seen in hyperthyroidism. It is also indicated for pain which often accompanies the above conditions.

4. The Prolactin Point (LTH)

This point mirrors the previously mentioned adrenal gland point on the edge of the tragus (concha-side). It is almost always painful in women with lactation complaints and those who suffer from mastopathy.

5. Parathormone Point (Parathyroid Point)

Needless to say, there is no superposed pituitary hormone which stimulates the parathyroid gland. The plasma-calcium level influences the parathyroid gland, hence regulating the parathormone secretion like a feedback mechanism. Accordingly, the parathormone point would not seem to fit in the hypophysis zone. However, it must be kept in mind that the auricular homunculus is nothing more than a synthetic figure created from individual observations, and an abstraction in its entirety *(W. Lang)*. It therefore follows that some points — especially those having significant actions — may by all means still be found at locations other than those where they would actually seem to fit.

I would like to cite the following study by *G. Kalcher,* as evidence of this point's action:

"The normal serum-calcium level is from 9.0 to 10.5 mg%. 55% of these are free, and hence, biologically active calcium ions.

The calcium content of extracellular fluid is subject to such precision regulation that one may speak of a 'biological constant'. The constancy of the serum calcium is maintained via a double feedback mechanism, the hormone, calcitonin, and the parathormone playing the most decisive roles. The skeleton serves as calcium depot from which calcium may be mobilized by hormonal influences when required.

Calcium's broad biological spectrum is well known. It follows that disturbances in calcium metabolism may be the cause of manifold types of clinical symptoms, of these, only increased neuromuscular excitability due to calcium deficiency being mentioned here.

Our patients' disorders were exclusively in the form of hypocalcemia, being as a rule of slight severity and having no signs of latent tetany. In view of the usually chronic course of illness of our sanatorium patients, the calcium deficiency appeared to be mainly the result of disturbed basic regulation and not of true calcium loss.

Having long been familiar with acupuncture's ability to influence the basic response, we forfeited oral parenteral calcium administration, and carried out a therapeutic trial using ear acupuncture of the parathyroid point.

The following test setup was chosen for the first investigation:

1. taking of blood samples and determination of the serum-calcium level
2. needling of the parathyroid point in cases having hypocalcemia. The stainless steel needle remained in position for 20 minutes.
3. renewed determination of serum calcium after 24 hours had elapsed.

Seven patients having hypocalcemia of low to moderate degrees of severity were investigated in this study. Twenty-four hours after acupuncture, the calcium level had reached the norm in six of these seven patients. The calcium level remained below 9.0 mg% in one patient. The calcium increase was greater in cases having had extremely low starting values than in those having had values only just under the norm. Values surpassing the norm were not observed.

In our opinion, this investigation gives evidence of the efficacy of ear acupuncture of the parathyroid point for hypocalcemia.

A second trial aimed at determining the point in time at which the effect took place and the duration of the latter.

Five patients were tested, a new model being used.

1. taking of blood samples and determination of calcium level
2. needling of the point and immediate renewed calcium level determination.
3. further measurements of serum calcium after 2 and 24 hours.

The values of these probands at the 24th hour were analogous with those changes observed in the initial investigation. In all patients, the time curve of the Ca values' rise had two peaks, the maximum peak being reached immediately following acupuncture, and the second after 24 hours. Control investigations carried out after one week or later showed normal values in all cases.

The next Table mathematically summarizes the results of these investigations:

F-Test		and		t-Test (Student)
H 12	before			after
x_2	8.17 mg %			9.37 mg %
s	0.5675			1.937
		F	= 3.457	
		p	< 0.01	
		s	= 0.459	
		D	= 1.20	
		t	= 2.614	
		p	< 0.01	

24 hours after needling, there has been a significant increase in the Ca^{++} level of an average of 1.2 mg %. The scatter of the values is significantly higher 24 hours after than prior to needling

Tab. 2: Comparison of Ca^{++} values before and 24 hours after acupuncture of the auricular parathyroid point after *NOGIER*.

That concludes the discussion of the projection of the hypophysis. I would like to stress that these reflex zones involve the hypophyseal projections only and not the reflex cartography of the endocrine glands. The latter shall be discussed later on.

C) The Projection of the Mesencephalon (Midbrain)

This projection lies in the foremost part of the inferior hemiconcha somewhat below the external auditory meatus. This area may correspond with the basal ganglia, as general reactions on **muscle tone** can be achieved via this projection (center of the musculature according to *Nogier*).

In particular, a point can be found in this area which has a distinct influence on **dysmenorrhoeic** complaints. This region should also be considered in cases of muscle tension, such as that often seen in the trapezial region.

Below the above-described point lies an area via which dyspareunia can be treated.

D) The Projection of the Spinal Cord

The reflex zone of the spinal cord projects to that portion of the helix margin which is innervated by the superficial cervical plexus. Hence, it extends from the Darwinian turbercle to the point of interesection of an imaginary line drawn from the O-point through the posterior antitragal groove with the margin of the helix. In accordance with the general hypothetical projection of a fetus lying upside down in the auricle, the segments of the coccygeal plexus lie below the Darwin point. The reflex zones of the corresponding segments then follow downwards. The termination of this zone at the helix-lobule angle represents the zone for the cervical plexus.

The projection of the **somatosensitive fibers** of the dorsal horn lie on the anterior side; that of the **somatomotor fibers** of the anterior horn on the dorsal side of the helix. Stimulating the corresponding region of the sensitive portions of the spinal cord influences certain disorders of sensibility and paresthesia which may appear in disturbances of peripheral nerves. Thus, for example, sensitive points will be found in the corresponding reflex zone of the affected segment in cases of herpes zoster. If these points are acupunctured with a gold needle and the O-point with a silver needle at the same time, the intolerable pain can often be eliminated.

In cases of poliomyelitis for example, points will be found in the motor zone on the dorsal surface of the helix which correspond with the paralyzed motor nerves. Needless to say, these points are only of diagnostic significance.

2. The Projection of the Autonomic System
(Sympathetic, Parasympathetic)

Anatomical Outline

The vegetative or autonomic nervous system innervates the smooth musculature of all organs and organic systems, the heart, the glands, and regulates the vital functions of respiration, circulation, digestion, metabolism, secretion, and reproduction.

It is an anatomic and functional unit which regulates the organic functions via inhibition or stimulation.

The two functional parts influence the functions of the internal organs antagonistically. They are:

The Sympathetic System and the Parasympathetic System

The center of regulation of both systems lies in the hypothalamus. Certain hypothalamic centers integrate all vegetative functions. These nuclei regulate the organism's vegetative functions by means of hormonal and neurosecretory mechanisms, as well as via nervous pathways. This is how the internal environment is regulated. Through the close connection between the hypothalamus and cerebrum, corresponding behavior patterns such as breathing reflexes, reproduction mechanisms, etc. are also released.

Anatomically, the two parts of the system are differentiated by the varying location of their cell bodies within the CNS and by the varying switching location of their peripheral processes.

The Sympathetic System

The nuclei of origin lie in the intermediolateral nucleus in the lateral horn of the spinal cord in the thoracic and upper lumbar region ($C_8 - L_3$). The sympathetic system's preganglionic fibers leave the spinal column through the anterior roots, and their switching location is found in the paravertebral sympathetic ganglia.

In the cervical region, the number of ganglia is reduced to 3 (stellate g., middle cervical g., and superior cervical g.); in the lumbar and sacral regions to 4 each.

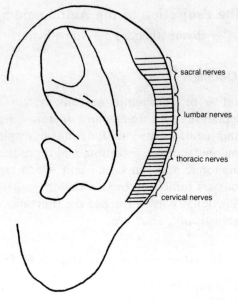

Fig. 22: The projections of the somatosensory spinal cord fibers.

The arrangement of the paravertebral ganglia is very precise in the thoracic region. Furthermore, there are connected sympathetic fibers arising from several segments which arrive at the prevertebral ganglia via the paravertebral, where their switching location is found.

In the cervical region these are the cardiac nerves; in the thoracic region, the pulmonary, and the greater and lesser splanchnic nerves; in the lumbosacral portion, the lumbar and sacral splanchnic nerves.

The prevertebral ganglia are arranged in large networks (pulmonary, cardiac, celiac, superior and inferior mesenteric, and hypogastric plexus).

The sympathetic nerve fibers for the head emerge from the spinal cord segments C_8—Th_2. Their synapse is in the superior cervical ganglion. They then accompany the large vessels of the head as periarterial networks, arriving at their effectors, such as the lacri-

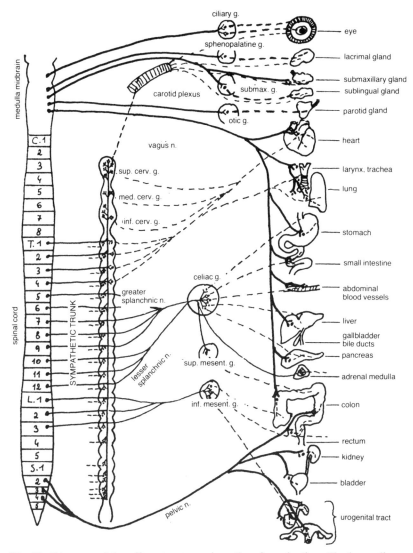

Fig. 23: Diagram of the efferent autonomic paths of conduction. The heavy lines represent parasympathetic fibers; the dotted lines, sympathetic (from *Youmans: Fundamentals of Human Physiology*, 2nd ed., Year Book, 1962)

mal and salivary glands, smooth muscles, and mucous membrane (external and internal carotid plexus, jugular plexus). The neck and throat region is supplied by the three cervical ganglia.

The fibrous networks of the body wall and the extremities emerge from the nuclei of Th_2-L_2.

The fibers for the arm arise mainly from the stellate ganglion; those for the leg traverse the sympathetic ganglia from L_4 to S_3. These only synapse when they have reached the prevertebral networks of this area.

The Parasympathetic System

In contrast to the sympathetic system, the switching locations of the parasympathetic system lie near the reacting organs.

In the head region, the fibers either join the cerebral nerves or travel independently (e. g. the vagus nerve). According to its nuclei of origin, the parasympathetic system can be subdivided into cranial and sacral parts.

The cranial part receives its fibers from cells of origin of the mesencephalon and rhombencephalon, which then join the oculomotor nerve, facial nerve, glossopharyngeal nerve, and vagus nerve. Peripherally, the preganglionic fibers in parasympathetic ganglia give rise to postganglionic neurons, which then travel partially with other cerebral nerves to the reacting organs.

The sacral cells of origin lie in the substantia intermedia centralis of the spinal cord. The preganglionic fibers form the pelvic splanchnic nerves and travel to the prevertebral plexus (superior and inferior hypogastric plexus, prostaticovesical or uterovaginal plexus). Here a partial synapse takes place; predominantly intramurally in the various pelvic organs. The fibers of the sacral parasympathetic system supply the pelvic viscera and the distal section of the large intestine starting at Cannon and Böhm's point. This point, which lies on the border of the distal third of the transverse colon, represents the innervation borderline between the cranial vagus and the sacral parasympathetic system.

No nuclei of origin of the parasympathetic system are contained in the middle portion of the lateral horn of the spinal cord.

a) The Projection of the Sympathetic Nuclei of Origin
(intermediolateral nuclei)

Accoding to *Nogier,* this zone is found in the concavity of the body of the helix and is bordered by 2 imaginary lines through the

O-point. One of these lines runs through the 12th thoracic verta-bra, the other through the posterior antitragal groove, and both in-tersect the margin of the helix.

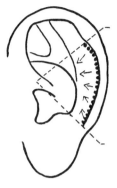

Fig. 24: The projection of the intermediolateral nuclei

b) The Projection of the Sympathetic Trunk

I have already mentioned that the projection of the paraverte-bral system lies parallel to the projection of the spinal column, in the groove of the anthelix which forms its border to the concha. Hence, it fills the narrow zone of the concha which is not inner-vated by the vagus.

Three ganglia are found in the cervical region:

1. the superior cervical ganglion

on the level of the 1st and 2nd cervical vertebrae.

2. the medial cervical ganglion

in front of the 3rd cervical vertebra.

These two ganglia are of little practical use. In contrast, the low-est of the 3 cervical ganglia offers us many therapeutic possibili-ties.

3. the inferior cervical ganglion

(stellate ganglion)

Its projection zone lies in front of the 7th cervical vertebra. Ana-tomically, this ganglion is the coordination site of all afferent and efferent sympathetic fibers of the upper fourth of the body. Thus, this zone will be measurable when, for example, the patient has suffered a **whiplash** in a car accident, spasms of the m. pectoralis minor, or cervical rib syndrome.

Since this ganglion also supplies the sympathetic plexus around the vertebral artery, this zone is effective for cervical migraine and Ménière's disease.

The thoracic ganglia are strictly arranged and lie in front of the projection of each corresponding vertebra. I would like to discuss two in particular:

1. The sympathetic fibers which travel to the **liver** are found on the level of the 5th and 6th thoracic vertebrae. This zone represents **the neural liver point.**

The organ projection will be discussed later on.

2. The sympathetic fibers of the **adrenal gland** lie on the level of the 12th thoracic vertebra. Here, please recall that the adrenal medulla basically represents a sympathetic ganglion.

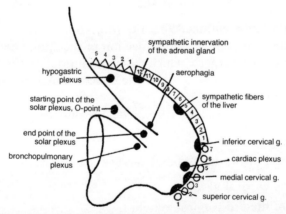

Fig. 25: The concha with the projection of the sympathetic trunk with its para and prevertebral ganglia

c) The Projection of the Prevertebral Ganglia

While the paravertebral ganglia are purely sympathetic, the prevertebral and periarterial ganglia are functionally mixed, that is, they contain predominantly parasympathetic parts. The united sympathetic nerve fibers from several segments synapse at this level where they also combine with the parasympathetic fibers to form the prevertebral plexus.

1. The Cardiac Plexus

The cardiac plexus is located immediately in front of the projection of the medial cervical ganglion, hence, on the level of the 3rd cervical vertebra. These two zones can be said to form a homogenous reflex region corresponding with *Nogier*'s "wonder point." This zone can influence certain types of hypertension. It is also sensitive to pressure in patients suffering from spasms or pain in the upper half of the body. The point is also of particular significance in all cases of vegetative regulatory disorders characterized by heart complaints. These particularly anxious patients, who suffer from sinus tachycardia, respiratory arrhythmia, and non-organic extrasystoles, should be treated via this area. *Nogier* also called this area the anxiety zone.

2. The Bronchopulmonary Plexus

The bronchopulmonary plexus lies on the level of the middle of the root of the helix, about 2—3 mm below an elevation which can always be distinctly felt, and which we call the plexus point, hence, on the upper border of the inferior hemiconcha. Bronchospastic conditions can be favorably influenced via this area.

3. The Solar Plexus

The solar plexus is formed by the interweaving of the celiac and superior mesenteric plexus. The anterior half of the root of the helix represents its reflex zone on the ear. Corresponding to the anatomic innervation, all spasms of the stomach, duodenum, jejunum, and ileum, ascending and transverse colon, the liver, gallbladder, and bile ducts, as well as the arteries of the abdominal cavity, can be influenced via this area.

Two points are of particular interest, whereby I must stress that in cases of spastic conditions in the abdomen, the entire zone must be examined for reflex points.

a) The O-Point

This point is found on the border of the root of the helix and the ascending branch of the helix in a groove running diagonally across the root. It is easy to find with the stirrup and can always be located electrically with the Punctoscope. Lytic treatment of all painful spasms of the viscera can be performed via this point. The unpleasant, involuntary contractions of the diaphragm (singultus/ hiccups), which may appear as a result of pressure from the stomach or liver, or following abdominal surgery, can also be favorably influenced via this point. Occasionally, it may be necessary to stimulate both O-points with an electrical stimulation device (see *Kampik* in "Akupunktur in Theorie und Praxis", No. 3, 1975).

Because of its mixed sympathetic and parasympathetic innervation, it should also be included in the therapy program in cases where extreme nervous tension has led to vegetative imbalance. Here, this point must always be acupunctured before the other points in the program.

If, however, unwanted vagosympathetic reactions have occured in the course of ear acupuncture treatment, the O-point should be acupunctured last in order to eliminate these disturbances.

Aside from these therapeutic possibilities, this point also affects the reactive ability of the entire auricle; you will sometimes observe patients on whose ears neither pressure-sensitive nor electrically measurable points can be found. This relatively rare absence of reflexes can be easily surmounted by acupuncturing the O-point with a gold needle. Vice-versa, hypersensibility of the ear can be normalized by acupuncturing the O-point with a silver needle. In both cases, point detection must be performed anew after a short period has elapsed.

Sometimes merely acupuncturing the O-point causes a change in the patient's state. A similar reaction is also seen when stimulation of well-chosen points has yielded no decisive results. Here, acupuncturing the O-point, which in such a case seems to be superior to the actually more suitable reflex points, is required to achieve the desired result.

Another interesting phenomenon in the auricle in regard to the O-point is the linear distribution of active characteristic points.

After an accurate examination of the auricle, you may sometimes observe that all the discovered points lie on one line which passes through the O-point. *Nogier* calls these "**line points.**"

If you extend this line to the margin of the ear, another active point may be found on this point of intersection. Stimulation of this margin point together with the O-point surpasses the effect of the points inbetween, and also reduces the number of needles required. The effect of these so-called "**ear margin points**" may be delayed, but is just as long-lasting.

In their study of the line and ear margin points, *Nogier* and his co-workers came across another very interesting phenomenon, which completed the "**ear geometry**". If two further straight lines are drawn from the discovered ear margin point at a 30° angle to the line ear margin point — O-point, two more very effective pressure-sensitive points may be found.

All these ear points should be used for chronic disorders of long standing when the normally located correspondence points have produced no satisfactory results.

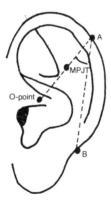

Fig. 26: Ear geometry. (Example: a case of chronic pain in the metacarpophalangeal joint of the thumb. An active point is found on the typical location (MPJT). If this point is connected to the O-point via an imaginary line which is then extendend to the margin of the ear, a new active point (A) can be found on this point of intersection. Sometimes another important point can be found. This point (B) then lies on the point of intersection of another line which traverses the margin of the ear and forms a 30° angle with the line O—A. Points such as these which are found through ear geometry are sometimes more effective than the typical correspondence point)

b) The Plexus Point

This point lies on a small elevation approximately in the middle of the root of the helix and can always be easily felt with the fingernail. It acts on the abdominal cavity. It is distinctly sensitive to pressure in all cases of intestinal pain and spasm, so that these complaints can be favorably influenced via this point. This point is also indicated for patients who have undergone surgery in the splanchnic region and complain of pain or dizziness.

At the base of this point towards the inferior and superior hemiconcha, two more points are found which are used for **aerophagia**.

4. The Hypogastric Plexus

With its mixed fibers, it supplies the descending colon, sigmoid, and rectum, the urogenital organs of the male (plexus vesicoprostaticus) and female (plexus uterovaginalis).

It is located on the ear in the foremost part of the superior hemiconcha between the projection of the bladder and the colon. The organs of this innervation region are treated via this area.

d) The Projection of the Parasympathetic System

Anyone who has used this method for some length of time agrees that the areas representing projections of the parasympathetic system are found in a narrow band lying in the transition area between the external auditory foramen and the inferior hemiconcha, partially including the beginning section of the auditory canal. This also coincides exactly with the corresponding anatomy, as the auricular ramus of the vagus arrives at the middle of the sharp edge of the external auditory meatus on the surface, supplying the concha, floor, and posterior wall of the external auditory meatus. It goes without saying that sharp borderlines of different areas cannot be drawn in such a small area, but rather, that smooth transitions probably exist, partially overlapping as well.

Indeed, this chapter clearly shows how new research of the reflex zones of the ear really is. That explains why results are constantly undergoing revision, extension, and modification.

For reasons pertaining to the history of the method, I would like to describe the development of the reflex locations of the cerebral nerves on the ear in chronological order.

About ten years ago, *Nogier* and *Bourdiol* placed the reflex zones of the nuclei of origin of the cranial parasympathetic system perimeatal, in the sharp edge of the external auditory meatus or oriented just slightly toward the concha. Shortly afterwards, they were moved to the periphery of the lobule, no explanatory data having been provided. Was this new location on the ear perhaps selected for "topographical" reasons only (spinal cord — medulla oblongata — pons — cranial nerve nuclei)? In my opinion, rapid development and the striving for constant renewal led to premature publication, neglecting the fact that the various zones on the lobule serve intensification of mental functional capacity.

I am also of the opinion that projections of cranial nerves cannot be found on the ear, not to mention these being divided into bulbar and peripheral parts. I feel that perimeatal reflex points can at best correspond with innervation areas of vegetative partial functions of cranial nerves.

Parasympathetic projections are found within a narrow band which is located at the transition from the external auditory foramen to the inferior hemiconcha, and partially includes the beginning portion of the auditory canal.

These perimeatal reflex zones are to be named only after the area on which they act. As they mainly correspond with the beginning portion of the digestive and respiratory tract, they shall be discussed in those sections.

The following is a simple list for learning purposes:

1. **The Rhinopharynx Zone**
   is located above the auditory meatus
2. **The Larynx Zone**
   extends downwards from the middle of the dorsal margin of the external auditory meatus to just above its lower border
3. **The Zone of Vagal Cardiac Regulation**
   lies in the lowest quarter and 2—3 mm behind the edge of the opening of the external auditory meatus
4. **The Zone of "Respiratory Automatics"**
   lies just above and behind the zone of cardiac regulation.

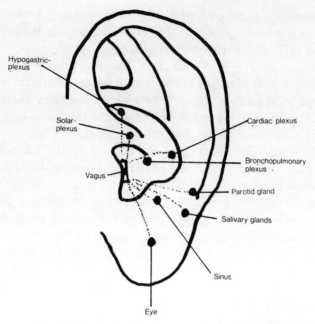

Fig. 27: The projection of the parasympathetic system

e) The Projection of the Thoracic Organs

1. The Heart

a) The Projection of the Heart

The projection of the heart is found on the level of the projection zone of the 4th and 5th thoracic vertebra on the dorsal part of the body of the anthelix corresponding to the region of the 2nd to 5th ribs. Active points may be observed here in cases of angina pectoris.

b) The Zone of Vagal Cardiac Regulation

There is a very vital point in the lowest dorsal quarter of the opening of the external auditory meatus, 2 to 3 mm behind its margin. Great caution must be taken when acupuncturing this point as the danger of syncope exists.

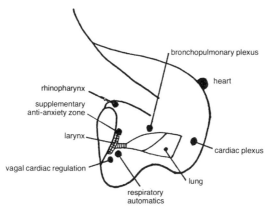

Fig. 28: Inferior hemiconcha with the projection of the thoracic organs

The area of the cardiac plexus corresponds rather with functional cardiac complaints and may represent the reflex zone of the carotid sinus.

The projection of the thoracic viscera (with the exception of the heart) is located on the vertical portion of the inferior hemiconcha. However, a small strip towards the root of the helix remains free. The esophagus projects into this area.

Hence, according to *Nogier*, **the representation of the diaphragm** is not the branch of the helix as stated by the Chinese, but rather begins below the O-point, and travels dorsally, leaving the root of the helix from which it is separated by the projection of the esophagus. At the level of the 3rd cervical vertebra, in front of the projection of the medial cervical ganglion, it forms a concave curve forwards and enters the superior hemiconcha in which it gradually approaches the anterior sharp margin of the anthelix. It reaches the latter on the level of the first portion of the projection of the lumbar vertebrae.

2. The Respiratory System

a) The Larynx Zone

This zone lies behind the lower third of the sharp margin of the auditory meatus. You will find points in this area in cases of changes in the boney larynx, hoarseness resulting from inflammation of the vocal cords, and dysphagia.

On the uppermost border of this area, towards the middle of the margin of the meatus, a point is found which combats anxiety. This area should be stimulated especially in cases of stagefright and fear of examinations.

b) The Projection of the Trachea

It adjoins the reflex zones for the larynx and vocal cords dorsally.

c) The Projection of the Lungs

This area fills almost the entire vertical surface of the inferior hemiconcha. Points in this region become active in patients with pulmonary disorders or bronchospastic conditions.

d) The Zone of "Respiratory Automatics" according to Nogier

This zone is found on the level of the lowest quarter of the sharp edge of the auditory meatus somewhat behind and above the zone of cardiac regulation. This zone is effective for all asthmatic complaints.

e) The Zone of the Bronchopulmonary Plexus

This zone has already been discussed in the chapter on the sympathetic system, but it should be mentioned again here. It lies approximately 2—3 mm below the plexus point in the uppermost part of the inferior hemiconcha and is also effective for bronchospastic conditions.

f) The Projection of the Digestive System

While the reflex cartography in the triangular fossa, the scapha, the anthelix, and the inferior hemiconcha is very distinct, two different reflex locations have been found in the superior hemiconcha for the organs of the visceral tract.

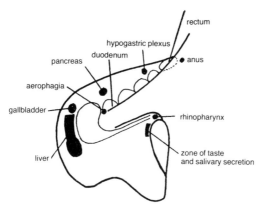

Fig. 29: The right superior hemiconcha with the **organ projection** of the gastro-intestinal tract

According to *Nogier,* the projection areas which adjoin the root of the helix correspond with the organs themselves, while the zones in the periphery of the superior hemiconcha correspond with the vegetative innervation of these organs. The latter are the result of investigations made by *Jarricot* et al.

Another possible explanation for the existence of two reflex locations for one organ in the concha may lie in the nature of the autonomic nervous system itself. The varying transmitting mechanisms between pre and postganglionic fibers of the sympathetic and parasympathetic system may provide the neuroanatomical explanation.

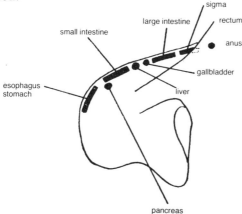

Fig. 30: The projection of the **vegetative innervation** of the abdominal viscera

This could explain why *Nogier's* visceral projections, which wind around the entire branch of the helix, may correspond with the sympathetic prevertebral ganglia or postganglionic neurons for each organ. This could be the case for the simple reason that from the O-point to the plexus point, the branch of the helix represents the solar plexus, that is, a nerve network in which the synapses of predominantly sympathetic fibers are found.

Hence, the reflex zones in the periphery of the superior hemiconcha correspond with the respective parasympathetic switching locations which lie in the immediate proximity of the reacting organ.

Bossy's neuroanatomical studies on the innervation of the concha confirm this. According to *Bossy,* the vagal innervation does not extend to the outer margin of the concha, but rather a small strip remains free. (The sympathetic trunk projects to this area.) The projection of the viscera was found to be within the vagal zone. I shall list both projection zones in the following sections.

After this brief hypothetical discussion, let us continue with the description of the locations of the individual sections of the digestive tract.

1. The Projection of the Rhinopharynx

This area lies immediately above the auditory meatus, under the roof formed above by the ascending branch of the helix and by the tragus anteriorly. It has a distinct influence on all forms of rhinitis, sinusitis, as well as on the olfactory sense.

2. The Zone for the Sense of Taste

This zone comprises a region in the upper quarter of the dorsal margin of the auditory meatus. This zone must be carefully examined in cases of impaired sense of taste.

3. The Esophagus

According to *Nogier,* the projection of the esophagus lies in the anterior upper part of the inferior hemiconcha commencing directly behind the above-described zones. Always travelling beneath the branch of the helix, it extends dorsally to approximately the level of the plexus point.

The neural location is found above the origin of the branch of the helix, just in front of the body of the anthelix, approximately on the level of the 4th—5th cervical vertebra.

Pain or spasm in the esophageal region can be influenced via this area.

4. The Stomach

According to *Nogier,* the stomach projects to the region adjoining the esophagus behind the origin of the root of the helix around which it winds. It covers most of the dorsal part of the superior hemiconcha.

The neural reflex zone adjoins that of the esophagus just in front of the dorsal border of the superior hemiconcha on the level of the lower cervical vertebra.

Here, the difference in the two locations in regard to diagnosis and therapy becomes evident for the first time. Active points are found in the organ zone in patients with vegetative disturbances suffering from stomach complaints with no significant clinical findings, stomach spasms, disturbances in acid secretion, or gastritis. Points in the neural zone are distinctly hypersensitive in cases of ulcers and carcinoma of the stomach.

5. The Duodenum

According to *Nogier,* the reflex zone of the duodenum lies in front of the margin of the branch of the helix facing the superior hemiconcha on the level of the plexus point. This point has already been described in the discussion of the plexus point and is effective in the treatment of aerophagia. It is also used to combat anxiety.

The neural projection of the duodenum and the entire small intestine projects to the same region of the superior hemiconcha, anterior to the anthelix, above the projection of the stomach, approximately on the level of the first thoracic vertebra.

6. The Small Intestine

According to *Nogier,* the representation of the small intestine entwines the projection of the stomach. *Bourdiol* is of the opinion that the entire convolution of the small intestine fills all the spaces in the superior hemiconcha.

7. The Colon

Nogier places the projection of the various viscera in that ear which corresponds with the anatomical location, that is, ipsilaterally. This can be better comprehended if you imagine a sagittal cut through the abdomen. Hence, you will find the following:

right ear
duodenum,
the right-sided portions of the
small intestine
ascending colon,
the right part of the transverse
colon,
the right lobe of the liver,
bile ducts,
pancreas.

left ear
stomach,
the left-sided portions of
the small intestine
the left lobe of the liver,
the left part of the transverse
colon,
the left flexure of the colon,
descending colon,
sigmoid.

The esophagus, rectum, and anus are found on both ears, as, anatomically speaking, they lie in the middle of the body.

According to *Nogier,* the projection of the colon in the ear itself lies in the lowest part of the superior hemiconcha along the root of the helix. It adjoins the projection of the stomach and extends from the plexus point to below the ascending branch of the helix. The projection of the rectum lies in the foremost angle of the concha towards the inner side of the ascending branch of the helix. Because of the fact that hyperplasia of the corpus cavernosum recti is the cause of hemorrhoids, it is not surprising that extremely active points are found here in such cases. Stimulation of this region on both ears achieves amazingly rapid alleviation of pain.

The anus lies in the extension of the projection of the rectum on the outer surface of the ascending branch of the helix.

Following the line of its previous projections forwards from the esophagus, stomach, and small intestine, you will find the neural projection of the large intestine on the level of the plexus point or the projection of the 11th and 12th thoracic vertebrae, commencing with the ascending colon and continuing with the transverse and descending colon to the foremost upper part of the concha. Here lies the reflex location of the rectum.

According to my practical experience, preference should be given to the organ projections especially because patients receiving auricular therapy have complaints of a predominantly functional, motor nature (irritable colon, spasms in cases of ulcerative colitis).

I observed in every case that both electrical examination of the ear and probe examination revealed points which corresponded with the site of the respective intestinal portion.

8. The Liver

According to *Nogier,* the projection of the liver parenchyma lies behind that of the stomach on the level of the 7th cervical vertebra. The zone is larger on the right ear than on the left. This location corresponds with Chinese reports which describe points in this zone in cases of swollen liver and cirrhosis of the liver.

Nogier describes another area for the liver, which, however, corresponds with its sympathetic innervation and lies on the level of the 5th—6th thoracic vertebrae in the uppermost part of the superior hemiconcha below the curve of the anthelix.

9. The Gallbladder

Its projection lies on the right ear only above the liver and behind the stomach toward the anthelix on the level of the 6th thoracic vertebra.

10. The Pancreas

According to *Nogier,* this projection is found on the right ear only. It lies above the projection of the duodenum.

The neural reflex zone is found adjoining the neural liver zone on the level of the 7th thoracic vertebra.

g) The Projection of the Peripheral Endocrine Glands

In the discussion of the reflex zone of the hypophysis, I have already mentioned the reflex locations of the central glandular regulation. In this chapter, I shall deal with the projections of the hypothalamic — hypophyseal reacting organs, in other words, the peripheral endocrine glands.

1. The Parathyroid Gland

Its projection lies in the angle formed by the anthelix and a line representing the extension of the upper margin of the root of the helix, hence, in the lowest dorsal corner of the superior hemiconcha somewhat in front of the location of the paravertebral ganglia.

Its effect is noteworthy in cases of muscle cramps as well as muscle tension.

2. The Thyroid

The thyroid projects to the level of the 6th and 7th cervical vertebrae somewhat in front of the projection of the stellate ganglion.

3. The Mammary Gland

The mammary gland is represented on the level of the 5th thoracic vertebra somewhat in front of the sympathetic trunk. It is the most important region for the female breast.

4. The Adrenal Gland

Corresponding to the histological stucture of the adrenal medulla, which actually represents a sympathetic ganglion in which the postganglionic neurons have lost their axons and have been transformed into secretory cells, its projection lies on the location of the sympathetic ganglion on the level of the 12th thoracic vertebra.

5. The Thymus

On the level of the 1st and 2nd thoracic vertebrae. This point must be included in the treatment of all types of allergies. It is usually acupunctured with a silver needle on the left and with a gold needle on the right.

When applying the points of the endocrine system for therapy, you must make sure that the patient's medical history is exact and that necessary laboratory tests are made. Only then will you be able to decide if therapy should be performed with points of the glandular projection or with those of hypophyseal glandular regulation.

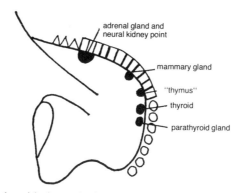

Fig. 31: The concha with the projection of the peripheral endocrine glands

Simultaneous stimulation of both will produce no positive results, as counter-regulation mechanisms are obviously called into action. Stimulation of the peripheral parts seems to inhibit the central effect.

85

h) The Projection of the Urogenital System

1. The Kidney

This organ also has two reflex areas. The reflex zone of the parenchyma lies on the inferior surface of the ascending branch of the helix at the level of the projection of the foot. The neural area is found (as also reported by the Chinese) in the superior hemiconcha on the level of the 12th thoracic vertebra, thus in the same zone in which the neural projection of the adrenal gland is found. In regard to the adrenal gland, the projection of the parenchyma coincides with the neural zone because embryologically, the adrenal medulla develops from the primitive ganglionic structure, that is, from the sympathetic formation. The size of the reflex area of the kidney parenchyma correlates with the organ (kidney). Thus, in cases of hydronephrosis for example, the reflex zone will be significantly enlarged.

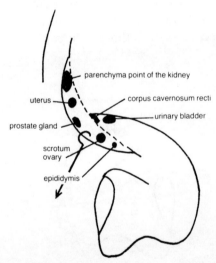

Fig. 32: The projection of the urogenital system (the ascending branch of the helix bent outwards)

A more important area is that of the ureter, which is found between the locations of the urinary bladder and the kidney.

In all cases of ureteral or renal colic, I have observed that the most active point is the area of the hypogastric plexus. I would like to repeat the description of its location here: It lies in the anterior section of the superior hemiconcha between the projection of the colon and that of the bladder. When examining this area in a patient with renal or ureteral colic, you will always find a point which is extremely painful on pressure and is almost always able to influence colic of the urogenital system.

2. The Urinary Bladder

It lies in the anterior upper part of the superior hemiconcha on the level of the 4th and 5th lumbar vertebrae.

3. The Urethra

The projection lies on the outer surface of the ascending branch of the helix and practically coincides with the location of the external genital organs.

4. The External Genital Organs

The reflex zones of the penis and clitoris are found on the outer surface of the ascending branch of the helix at the level of the lower crus of the anthelix.

5. Just below these zones and somewhat above the anterior notch, lies a zone which is able to increase the libido. *Nogier* named it **the Bosch Point** after the picture of the ear in Hieronimus *Bosch's* triptych "The Garden of Delights".

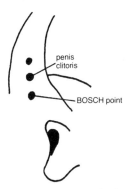

Fig. 33: The ascending branch of the helix with the projection of the external genitals

6. The projections of the **scrotum, epididymis, and ovary** lie on the inner surface of the ascending branch of the helix immediately after it emerges from the concha.

7. The Prostate Gland and the Uterus

Also on the inner surface of the ascending branch of the helix on the level of the lower crus of the anthelix.

3. Special Zones and Points

a) The Tragus

The tragus is the skin-covered piece of cartilage which hangs over the external auditory meatus and whose wide base joins the cheek. The base can be distinctly recognized especially in older persons by a vertical furrow. Corresponding points project to the base.

The tragus represents the anterior-posterior midline of the body, hence, corresponds with Tou Mo and Jenn Mo in classical acupuncture. Of particular importance is whether the patient is left or right-handed.

Thus, for example, the right tragus of a right-handed individual corresponds with Jenn Mo, or Conception Vessel, and in the left-handed patient with Tou Mo or Pilot Vessel. I shall take a **right-handed** subject as an example in describing the points lying in this region.

The right tragus represents Jenn Mo or the anterior midline. Accordingly, we find points on the previously mentioned line which correspond with the viscera in the sequence found when the body is turned upside-down.

Hence, the points for regulation of urogenital function correspond with the upper region. Continuing caudally, we find the points of the abdominal, then the thoracic region, and on the bottom the throat.

On **the left tragus,** which corresponds with Tou Mo, or the dorsal midline, the coccyx is found in the uppermost section of the furrow of the tragus, and the area of the gingiva (PV 27) on the lower end of the furrow.

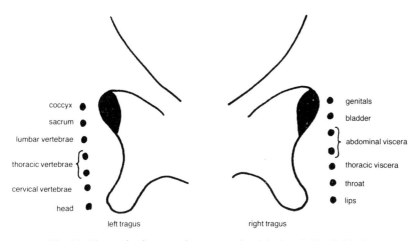

Fig. 34: The projections on the tragus of a right-handed individual

Thus, in a right-handed individual, the furrow of the right tragus regulates the vegetative functions of the viscera, while the furrow of the left tragus acts particularly on the skeletal system, ligaments, and muscles.

These zones must be systematically examined in cases of medial and bilateral pain in the region of the spinal column with its ligamentous system, the paravertebral muscles of the back, and the viscera.

Bourdiol assumes that the furrow of the tragus may correspond with the commissural pathways of the cerebral fibrous systems, that is, fibrous systems which connect the same cortical areas of both hemispheres.

b) The Allergy Point

This point lies somewhat in front of the highest point of the body of the helix.

It is easy to find if you bend the entire auricle forwards. A small triangular groove on the upper edge of the auricle is then formed at the tip of which the point lies. It corresponds with the point 10 outside of the meridians and is effective in treatment of allergies.

c) The Darwin Point

This point lies on the level of the Darwinian tubercle in a transverse groove on the helix which is located most easily with the "stirrup". According to *Nogier,* this groove represents a border zone between the innervation of the trigeminal nerve and the cervical plexus, hence it is very important.

This point was found empirically and is to be used for all complaints of the lower extremities.

d) General Tonification Point

This point lies just above the border between the lower and median thirds of the upper crus of the anthelix, oriented somewhat towards the triangular fossa. A Chinese point (Shen-Men, Gate of the Gods, No. 55) is found at the locus at which vessels from the auricule's medial side traverse to the lateral side, breaking through the auricular cartilage. With this point, any action set via the ear may be intensified by stimulating the abundant vascular nerves (sympathetic).

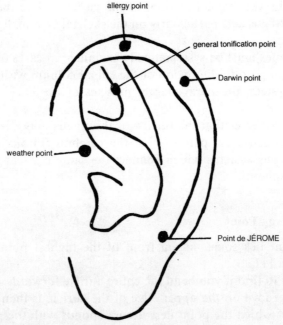

Fig. 35: Special points

e) The Weather Point

There are actually several points which are found in persons who are sensitive to weather conditions. They are found on the ascending branch of the helix where it meets the skin of the face, mainly on the right ear.

These points are especially important in the treatment of complaints such as angina pectoris, headache, or migraines which increase or appear during certain weather conditions.

f) Sleep Points

1. The *Point de Jérome* has already been mentioned and is also called *the relaxation point*. It lies exactly on the point of intersection of an imaginary line drawn from the O-point through the posterior antitragal groove with the transition point of the margin of the helix with the lobule, somewhat towards the edge of the ear.

It is indicated for patients who have difficulty in falling asleep, and is usually acupunctured with a gold needle.

2. Another important point which is used for sleep disturbances lies on the medial surface of the auricle corresponding to the relaxation point.

g) Psychologically Effective Points

1. The Anti-Fear Zone

The unpleasant sensation accompanying premonition of danger or mishap without marked vegetative reactions projects to the anterior, lower part of the earlobe in the region of the zone of the limbic cortex. In right-handed subjects, this fear projects to the right ear only. If, however, the fear is connected with strong vegetative reactions (palpitations, perspiration, and, especially, intestinal disorders), the root of the helix in the region of the plexus point must be examined.

2. The Anti-Aggression Zone

This zone lies directly above the previously described zone on the point of intersection of a vertical line through the anterior border of the intertragic notch with a horizontal line through the angle helix — lobule.

This area, too, is found on the right ear in right-handed subjects (and on the left ear in left-handed subjects).

The scale of emotions which may be treated via this area ranges from simple antagonism, hate, and maliciousness to the state in which an individual "contemplates violent acts and begins to plan them". In the latter case, a zone can even be found on the medial surface of the auricle corresponding to the anterior aggression area *(Nogier)*.

3. The "Psychosomatic Point"
(R-Point according to *Bourdiol*)

This point lies in front of the ascending branch of the helix on the spot where the lower border of the branch of the helix meets with the upper point of fusion of the helix with the skin of the face.

This point may be acupunctured outside or inside. In the latter case, the needle is inserted into the concavity of the groove of the helix on the level of the projection of the coccygeal bone. The tip of the needle is advanced forwards horizontally.

This point corresponds with the point "autonomic nervous system" on Chinese ear charts, which, however, do not give its exact location. Nevertheless, it is acupunctured in China in the above-described manner.

In cases of psychosomatic illness, this point is acupunctured in right-handed persons on the right with a silver needle and on the left with a gold needle. In cases having hallucinations, the metals are reversed.

This point must be included in the treatment of all psychosomatic disorders, such as bronchial asthma, nervous dyspepsia, peptic or duodenal ulcers, ulcerative colitis, and nervous heart conditions.

Bourdiol also mentions this point's psychoanalytical significance, as stimulation may also release repressed experiences.

In a right-handed patient, the point on the right is sedated (silver) and the point on the left tonified (gold).

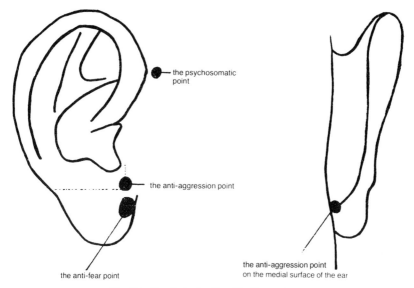

the psychosomatic point

the anti-aggression point

the anti-fear point

the anti-aggression point
on the medial surface of the ear

Fig. 36: Psychologically effective points

4. The Zones on the Medial Surface of the Auricle

Reflex zones which correspond to those on the lateral surface of the auricle are also found on the medial surface.

Because this surface is smaller, the zones are crowded together, hence, for a better overall view, only the projections of the individual body regions shall be presented at first. Just as on the lateral side, they are separated by the characteristics of the relief, which however, demonstrates the opposite characteristic (like a photo negative) (a fold on the lateral surface corresponds with a groove on the medial surface).

For study purposes, the anatomic names shall be maintained.

1. The Projection of the Somatomotor Roots of the Spinal Cord

This is represented by the outermost border of the edge of the auricle and extends from the level of the Darwinian tubercle to a little above the angle helix — lobule.

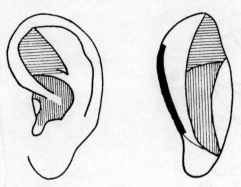

Fig. 37: Comparison of the zones of the lateral and medial surfaces of the auricle

≡ = zone of the lower extremity
☐ = zone of the upper extremity
⫶⫶⫶ = visceral zone
■ = zone of the somatomotor roots of the spinal cord

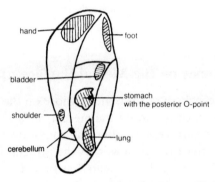

Fig. 38: Some important zones on the medial projection surface of the auricle

2. The Projection of the Upper Extremities

This projection adjoins the motor spinal cord zone as far as the groove of the anthelix, whereby the boundary of the upper third is represented by the groove of the upper crus of the anthelix, and in the middle and lower third, by the groove of the body of the anthelix. Corresponding to the lateral side of the auricle, the points for the fingers are found in the upper region and those for the shoulder in the lower region.

3. The Projection of the Viscera

The outer boundary of this area is represented by the groove of the anthelix; the upper border by the groove of the lower crus of the anthelix. The sulcus retroauricularis represents the inner boundary.

The bladder projects to the upper, inner part; the lung to the lower, inner part. The remaining surface represents the projection of the gastrointestinal tract, whereby the stomach comprises the middle portion of the entire zone.

The posterior O-point is also found here opposite the plexus point of the root of the helix. Together with the anterior O-point, it has a favorable influence on aerophagia.

4. The Projection of the Lower Extremities

The zone which represents this projection is almost triangular and fills the surface which lies above the visceral zone and behind the zone of the upper extremities.

Indications

The areas on the medial surface of the auricle and their maximum points mainly serve intensification of the points stimulated at the corresponding loci on the lateral surface. They should be examined and included in therapy especially of any chronic painful conditions in joints, as well as those conditions in which pain is related to movement.

Should both surfaces of the ear be treated simultaneously, we recommend using precious metal needles. The metal used on the medial side should contrast: In case of pain caused by movement, for example, a silver needle should be inserted in the lateral side, and a gold needle in the medial side. The potential difference between gold and silver thus produced is evidently the cause of the intensified effect.

5. The Combination of Ear and Body Acupuncture

Just as erroneous as the belief that body acupuncture (BA) is the only conservative Chinese therapy is the notion that ear acupuncture (EA) alone is always sufficient. Traditional Chinese therapy consisted of a combination of acupuncture, massage, breathing and concentration exercises, and administration of medicinal herbs. In recent years, ear acupuncture has also been included.

In over ten years of practicing acupuncture, I have, as a rule, been using a combination of ear and body acupuncture.

Approximately 1,550 patients having complaints of the large joints, part of whom come to my office and part of whom come to the outpatient service of the Ludwig Boltzmann Acupuncture Institute, shall serve to illustrate the different effects.

The case material with which we are confronted may be considered as having poor prognoses, if not even as being a negative selection in view of the majority's already having undergone unsuccessful treatment for many years.

Analgesic consumption was taken as objective parameter of the therapy's efficacy, as in many cases, there was a conspicuous discrepancy between the patient's reports and the objectively raised findings.

Total:	1,550 patients
of these	525 had complaints of the knee
	441 had complaints of the hip
	326 had complaints of the shoulder
	358 had complaints of the elbow

No. of Patients	Ear			Body			Ear and Body		
Knee 525	175	86	(49 %)	196	133	(68 %)	154	111	(72 %)
Hip 441	132	32	(24 %)	147	40	(27 %)	162	52	(32 %)
Shoulder 326	109	74	(68 %)	98	70	(71 %)	119	98	(82 %)
Elbow 258	99	53	(54 %)	72	45	(62 %)	8	65	(75 %)

Tab. 3: Comparison of the positive results of treatment of various joints with ear acupuncture, body acupuncture, and combined ear and body acupuncture

Knee 525		rapid short-term		slow longer-lasting improvement		no	
ear acupuncture	175	82	(47 %)	4	(2 %)	89	(51 %)
body acupuncture	196	8	(4 %)	125	(64 %)	63	(32 %)
E & B	154			111	(72 %)	43	(28 %)

Tab. 4: Results of treatment of disorders of the joint of the knee

shoulder 326		rapid short-term		slow longer-lasting improvement		no	
ear acupuncture	109	73	(67 %)	1	(1 %)	35	(32 %)
body acupuncture	98	12	(12 %)	58	(59 %)	28	(29 %)
E & B	19			98	(82 %)	21	(18 %)

Tab. 5: Results of treatment of disorders of the shoulder joint

hip 441		rapid short-term		slow longer-lasting improvement		no	
ear acupuncture	132	30	(23 %)	1	(1 %)	101	(76 %)
body acupuncture	147	7	(5 %)	32	(22 %)	108	(73 %)
E & B	162			52	(32 %)	110	(68 %)

Tab. 6: Results of treatment of disorders of the hip joint

elbow 258		rapid short-term		slow longer-lasting improvement		no	
ear acupuncture	99	51	(52 %)	2	(2 %)	46	(46 %)
body acupuncture	72	3	(4 %)	42	(58 %)	27	(38 %)
E & B	87			65	(75 %)	22	(25 %)

Tab. 7: Results of treatment of disorders of the elbow joint

Following EA, the responses observed of the different joints vary (Tab. 3). The shoulder joint appears to react best (68 %), followed by the elbow (54 %) and knee joint (49 %). Least responsive was the hip joint (24 %). These results, which are unusually positive for the pathological-anatomical substrate, are nevertheless subject to limitation, as the effects are only short-term, manifesting themselves as a rule immediately after treatment, lasting, however, only a few days. Repeated application of auricular therapy leads to only an insignificant prolongation of the post-therapeutic pain alleviation.

Nevertheless, the immediate effect greatly impresses the patient and prompts him to place his trust in a treatment form which is, in most cases, unfamiliar. In some cases, usually acutely appearing joint afflictions caused, for example, by extreme strain, or pain resulting in immobilization of the joint, ear acupuncture may achieve not only an immediate effect, but one of long duration as well. Cases such as these do not, however, appear in the foregoing statistics.

Body acupuncture alone produces similar results. Here too, the hip joint responds least (27 %). Favorable results may be observed in cases of disorders of the shoulder (71 %), knee (68 %), and elbow (62 %) joints. With only a few exceptions in which an immediate effect is seen, body acupuncture seems to call forth a slow, gradual effect (Tab. 4—7). The effect may take several hours, days, or even several sessions to manifest itself.

The results are, however, of accordingly longer duration. We have observed cases being free of complaints for 3—4 months or having pain reduced to a tolerable degree for a longer period of time.

Patients who have received a combination of ear and body acupuncture provide the most impressive results. It appears that auricular therapy not only effectively bridges body acupuncture's ineffective interval, but also has an intensifying action (Tab. 3—7).

Guidelines for Therapy

1. Ear Acupuncture is not the only therapeutic method at your disposal

Supplement auricular therapy with conventional or homoeopathic medication, osteopathic manipulation, physical medicine, massage, etc.

Do not hesitate to apply substitutive therapy for anacidity or absence of enzymes.

2. Case History

The patient's case history must be taken down conscientiously. You must be able to listen to the patient. Important clues for therapy may be overlooked if you do not allow the patient to render a complete report about his condition and complaints.

Pay attention to seemingly unimportant details.

Your questions should always be direct in order to establish the causal genesis of the disorder.

Always consider the possibility of the disorder being psychosomatic.

Ask the patient whether he has scars on his body in order to detect possible fields of disturbance which may hinder the therapeutic effect.

3. Clinical Tests

Have X-rays made if indicated. Have laboratory tests carried out and obtain a specialist's opinion if necessary.

Patients often bring laboratory findings when they come for their first treatment with the most important items missing (i. e. blood sugar content, urological findings).

Clinical examination also includes having the patient demonstrate which movements cause pain and to which area it projects (for example in cases of pain in the extremities and thorax). You may then discover that the painful region described in the medical history does not at all coincide with the basic region, but rather represents the effect of pain radiation. This is also important for testing the treatment's effect.

4. Thorough Inspection of the Auricle

A magnifying glass should be used at times. Reddened point-formed or thickened areas, scales, or even ulcers may be discovered. Be sure you have good light.

5. Examination of the Auricle

Use a probe, bellied bougie, or an electrical device.

Remember that the point locations may vary due to variations of the ear relief. When locating points, always take basic connections regarding the appearance of the disorder into consideration, for example, asthma or joint complaints which first appeared during menopause. Examine the prefrontal zone in cases of chronic painful conditions and also if the patient is aggressive. Do not forget to examine the medial surface of the auricle and margin points.

6. Needle Insertion

Carefully cleanse the auricle with alcohol before every treatment. Use sterilized needles only.

There are no standard "recipes" in ear acupuncture! Stimulate only those points which you have found during your examination.

A small number of needles is often sufficient to produce decisive results.

Pay attention to the patient's "grimaces". Remember that ear acupuncture is a reflex therapy.

I am of the opinion that therapy via the auricle has only been successful when the peripheral complaints, such as pain or cramps, are alleviated immediately after the points have been needled.

The needles must not be inserted too deeply, that is, not through the cartilage, and not too superficially. The needles may also be inserted at an angle to keep them from falling out prematurely. This is indicated especially when vibratory or electrical stimulation is used.

A favorable action can be achieved if you rotate the needle once clockwise and once counterclockwise when inserting it.

You will also achieve better results if you have the patient take a deep breath while inserting the needle.

If the peripheral complaints increase, change needles immediately, i. e. replace a gold needle with a silver needle.

7. The Individual Treatment Period

In general, the needles are left in position for 15—20 minutes.

I have found premature removal of the needles immediately after the desired effect has taken place to be ineffective.

Always watch for bleeding after the needle has been removed. It only appears after a latency period of several seconds. If bleeding occurs, dab the area lightly and do not apply pressure. This avoids formation of a bruise.

8. The Frequency of Treatments

Two to three treatments per week are indicated for acute disorders. Chronic disorders require treatment only once a week. However, the frequency of treatments always depends on the patient's reaction. It is quite possible that one treatment alone may achieve long-term results.

9. Reactions

I have already mentioned the immediate disappearance of complaints within a matter of seconds.

However, you will also have patients whose complaints subside only gradually from treatment to treatment. This is usually the case in disorders of the visceral tract.

Particularly sensitive patients may experience worsening of their complaints the day after the first treatment. However, this should be evaluated as a positive reaction, as it generally tends to subside rapidly and, to a certain extent, initiates the healing phase.

Cases which are resistant to therapy may have an undiscovered field of irritation or more extensive anatomic alterations. Here, I am thinking mainly of hernias of the intervertebral disks.

However, even in cases having a severe lesion of this type, correct therapy may eliminate pain for a short time, indeed, the accompanying sensory disturbances may also disappear. However, the old complaints soon return.

Hence, with auricular diagnosis, you may discover, for example, a herniated nucleus pulposus, which will usually be clinically verified. Fields of irritation can be eliminated by means of neural therapy or body acupuncture.

Syncope may occur. The best way to avoid it is to have the patient lie down during the treatment.

As a rule, the first treatment should be performed with the patient lying down. Never acupuncture ear points during a myocardial infarction, asthma or angina pectoris attack. Do not stimulate spontaneously painful points, as unpleasant circulatory reactions may result.

Should syncope occur, I recommend removing all needles immediately. Lay the patient flat and needle the reliable acupuncture points P 9, H 9, or PV 25 (on the border between the upper and middle thirds of the philtrum).

10. Combining Auricular Therapy and Classical Acupuncture

The combination of auricular therapy and classical acupuncture can bring about very favorable results, indeed, an intensified effect is often observed. Therefore, I usually proceed by using auricular therapy first for chronic disorders. If positive results have been achieved, but some symptoms still remain, I then employ body acupuncture, thus achieving further improvement, if not complete rehabilitation. The sequence may also be reversed, however, do not forget that ear points only manifest themselves when painful or pathological conditions exist in the periphery. Therefore, they are found more easily when the complaints are intense. If the peripheral disorders have been reduced through classical acupuncture to such an extent that only slight complaints remain, the points on the ear will be difficult to locate. For acute disorders such as those of the spinal column and the paravertebral muscles, for example, I use ear acupuncture first as a rule for the simple reason that the patient will only be able to move and place himself on the examination table properly after the needles have been inserted into the ear. Here, I make an exception and acupuncture the ear points while the patient is still sitting or standing. I have never seen a patient with pain so severe as in acute lumbago collapsing when needled.

This sequence is also advantageous for purely technical reasons, as manipulation of the ear is more difficult if, for example, the patient is lying prone. Therefore, I find it incomprehensible that some authors recommend applying ear acupuncture after body acupuncture.

If you follow these guidelines, I am certain that you will find ear acupuncture to be a valuable supplement to the therapeutic methods at your disposal, and that it will bring you much satisfaction and positive results.

References

Bischko, J.: An Introduction to Acupuncture. Karl F. Haug Publishers, Heidelberg 1978.

Bourdiol, R. J.: Congress in Freudenstadt, 1969 and 1972.

Bourdiol, R. J.: Ear Acupuncture Course. Congress in Freudenstadt 1971.

Bourdiol, R. J.: Das periphere autonome Nervensystem in der Aurikulomedizin. Akupunkturarzt 6/7 and 8/9 (1975) 10/11 (1976).

Forssmann and Heym: Grundriß der Neuroanatomie. Springer-Verlag, Heidelberg 1979.

Ganong, W. F.: Medizinische Physiologie, Springer-Verlag, Heidelberg 1979.

Huard, P., Wong, M.: Chinesische Medizin. Kindler, München 1968.

Jarricot, H., Wong, M.: De l'Auriculothérapie, Meridiens 21–22 (1973).

Kalcher, G.: Normalization of the Blood Calcium Level by Ear Acupuncture, Congress Proceedings of the Second French, Italian, and Austrian Congress on Acupuncture and Auricular Therapy, Vienna 1975 (Ed.: *J. Bischko*), Egermann Publishers, Vienna, p. 189.

Kiszel, S.: personal communication.

König, G., Wancura, I.: Einführung in die chinesische Ohrakupunktur. 6. Aufl., Karl F. Haug Verlag, Heidelberg 1978.

Kropej, H.: Ohrakupunktur bei Ellbogenschmerz. Orthopädische Praxis 10, 10. 1980.

Kropej, H.: Die Rolle der Ohrakupunktur bei der Behandlung von Gelenkserkrankungen. Erfahrungsheilkunde 28 (1979) Heft 3.

Kropej, H.: Die Nichtbeachtung der Differentialdiagnose als Ursache des Versagens in der Akupunktur. Erfahrungsheilkunde 28 (1979) Heft 4.

Lang, W.: Akupunktur und Nervensystem. 2. Aufl., Karl F. Haug Verlag, Heidelberg 1976.

Mumenthaler, M.: Neurologie. Georg Thieme Verlag, Stuttgart 1979.

Nogier, P. F. M.: Traité d'Auriculothérapie. Maisonneuve, Geneva 1969.

Nogier, P. F. M.: Die Anatomie der Reflexzentren der Wirbelsäule. Akupunkturarzt (1974) 2.

Nogier, P. F. M.: Ohrgeometrie. Akupunkturarzt (1974) 3.

Nogier, P. F. M.: Psychotrope Punkte. Akupunkturarzt (1976) 12/13.

Plastic Ear Model

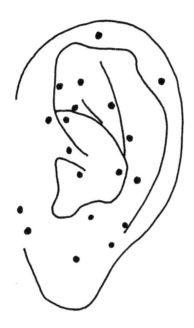

MD Helmut Kropej

*With the most important points of
ear acupuncture. Plastic model
and register of 4 pages.*

ISBN 3-7760-0835-0

*Karl F. Haug Publishers
P. O. Box 102840 · 6900 Heidelberg
Germany*

Plate of Ear Acupuncture

MD Georg König and
MD Ingrid Wancura

5th edition, 1990.
Coloured plate.
Size 24 × 34 inches.

The plate shows the auricle in a plastic
way. The ear points are numbered and
coloured to help the beginners. A sketch
of anatomy and of chinese organ-projec-
tion completes the plate.

Karl F. Haug Publishers
P. O. Box 102840
6900 Heidelberg
Germany

An Introduction to Acupuncture

By Prof. Johannes Bischko MD

Volume 1
2nd revised and enlarged English Edition.
124 pages, 18 figures, bound.

This concise and highly acclaimed book for the study of acupuncture (original German-language version already in its 14th edition) by the world-famous acupuncture expert *Johannes Bischko* provides the Western-trained physician with the foundations for the practical application of acupuncture.

Contains:
The most simple forms of acupuncture and the points they require
Energy and the meridians
The different types of points and their scientific explanation
Manipulation of neurotransmitters via acupuncture
The pulse diagnosis
The technique of acupuncture and the reactions it causes
Indications for acupuncture
The location and symptoms of the most important acupuncture points

The indications and points are cataloged in a comprehensive manner, which will serve the physician as an indispensable reference book for many years to come.

Karl F. Haug Publishers
P. O. Box 10 28 40
6900 Heidelberg
Germany

Einführung in die chinesische Ohrakupunktur

Von Dr. med. Georg König und Dr. med. Ingrid Wancura

9. Auflage, 144 Seiten, 59 Abbildungen, kartoniert.

Die Ohrakupunktur dient nur zu einem kleinen Teil der Behandlung von Ohrkrankheiten. Fast alle Erkrankungen, die der Akupunktur zugänglich sind, können gleichfalls auch durch Reizung bestimmter Punkte von der Ohrmuschel aus behandelt werden. Das gilt nicht nur für therapeutische Zwecke, sondern auch für die Operationsanalgesie. Die Autoren beschreiben bewußt nur die chinesische Ohrakupunktur, da über diese im Westen noch fast keine Veröffentlichung vorliegt.

Karl F. Haug Verlag
Postfach 10 28 40
W-6900 Heidelberg